D0908781

Tardive Dyskinesia: Biological Mechanisms and Clinical Aspects

Progress in Psychiatry

David Spiegel, M.D.,
Series Editor

Tardive Dyskinesia: Biological Mechanisms and Clinical Aspects

Edited by
Marion E. Wolf, M.D.
Aron D. Mosnaim, Ph.D.

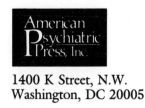

American Psychiatric Press, Inc.

1400 K Street, N.W.
Washington, DC 20005

Copyright © 1988 American Psychiatric Press, Inc.
ALL RIGHTS RESERVED
Manufactured in the United States of America
First Edition   88 89 90 91 5 4 3 2 1

The paper used in this publication meets the minimum requirements of American National Standard for Information Sciences—Permanence of Paper for Printed Library Materials, ANSI Z39.48-1984.   ∞™

Library of Congress Cataloging-in-Publication Data

Tardive dyskinesia: biological mechanisms and clinical aspects/ edited by Marion E. Wolf, Aron D. Mosnaim.
    p. cm.—(The Progress in psychiatry series)
    Includes bibliographies.
    ISBN O-88048-176-5 (alk. paper)
    1. Tardive dyskinesia.   I. Wolf, Marion E., 1945–
    .   II. Mosnaim, Aron D., 1940–   .   III. Series.
RC394.T37T364 1988   88-14590
616.8'3—dc19   CIP

Contents

Contributors

Phyllis E. Amabile, J.D., M.D.
Isaac Ray Center, Section of Psychiatry and the Law, Department of
Psychiatry, Rush-Presbyterian-St. Luke's Medical Center, Chicago,
Illinois

Sofia Avissar, Ph.D.
Ida and Solomon Stern Psychiatry Research Unit, Beer Sheva Mental
Health Center and Ben Gurion University of the Negev, Beer Sheva,
Israel

L. Jarrett Barnhill, M.D.
Department of Psychiatry, Biological Sciences Research Center,
University of North Carolina, Chapel Hill, North Carolina

Robert H. Belmaker, M.D., Ph.D.
Ida and Solomon Stern Psychiatry Research Unit, Beer Sheva Mental
Health Center and Ben Gurion University of the Negev, Beer Sheva,
Israel

Lise Belzile, R.N.
Douglas Hospital Centre and McGill University, Verdun, Quebec,
Canada

Richard L. Borison, M.D., Ph.D.
Department of Psychiatry, Augusta V.A. Medical Center and
Medical College of Georgia, Augusta, Georgia

Zachary Bregman, M.D.
Beth Israel Medical Center, New York, New York

Phil Brown, Ph.D.
Brown University, Providence, Rhode Island and Harvard Medical
School Program in Psychiatry and the Law, Massachusetts Mental
Health Center, Boston, Massachusetts

Yves Camille, M.D.
Douglas Hospital Centre and Department of Psychiatry, McGill University, Verdun, Quebec, Canada

James L. Cavanaugh, Jr., M.D.
Isaac Ray Center, Section of Psychiatry and the Law, Department of Psychiatry, Rush-Presbyterian-St. Luke's Medical Center, Chicago, Illinois

Timothy J. Crow, Ph.D., F.R.C.Psych.
Division of Psychiatry, Clinical Research Centre, Northwick Park Hospital, Harrow, England

Michael Davidson, M.D.
Department of Psychiatry, Bronx V.A. Medical Center, Bronx, New York and New York State University School of Medicine, New York, New York

Bonnie M. Davis, M.D.
Department of Psychiatry, Bronx V.A. Medical Center, Bronx, New York and New York State University School of Medicine, New York, New York

Kenneth L. Davis, M.D.
Department of Psychiatry, Bronx V.A. Medical Center, Bronx, New York and New York State University School of Medicine, New York, New York

Nicholas DeMartines, M.D.
Department of Psychiatry, Augusta V.A. Medical Center and Medical College of Georgia, Augusta, Georgia

Johans A. Den Boer, M.D.
Department of Biological Psychiatry, Utrecht University Hospital, Utrecht, The Netherlands

Joseph DeVeaugh-Geiss, M.D.
Clinical Research Section, Ciba-Geigy Corporation, Summit, New Jersey

Bruce I. Diamond, Ph.D.
Department of Psychiatry, Augusta V.A. Medical Center and Medical College of Georgia, Augusta, Georgia

Everett H. Ellinwood, Jr., M.D.
Department of Psychiatry, Duke University Medical Center, Durham, North Carolina

Thomas N. Ferraro, Ph.D.
Department of Neurology, Thomas Jefferson University, Philadelphia, Pennsylvania

William M. Glazer, M.D.
Department of Psychiatry, School of Medicine, Yale University, New Haven, Connecticut

C. Thomas Gualtieri, M.D.
Department of Psychiatry, Biological Sciences Research Center, University of North Carolina, Chapel Hill, North Carolina

Lars M. Gunne, M.D.
Psychiatric Research Center, Ulleraker Hospital, University of Uppsala, Uppsala, Sweden

Theodore A. Hare, Ph.D.
Department of Pharmacology, Thomas Jefferson University, Philadelphia, Pennsylvania

Per E. Johansson, M.D.
Psychiatric Research Center, Ulleraker Hospital, University of Uppsala, Uppsala, Sweden

Richard S. E. Keefe
Department of Psychiatry, Bronx V.A. Medical Center, Bronx, New York

William C. Koller, M.D., Ph.D.
Department of Neurology, University of Kansas Medical Center, Kansas City, Kansas

K. R. Rama Krishnan, M.D.
Department of Psychiatry, Duke University Medical Center, Durham, North Carolina

Edward D. Levin, Ph.D.
Psychiatric Research Center, Ulleraker Hospital, University of Uppsala, Uppsala, Sweden

Miklos F. Losonczy, M.D., Ph.D.
Department of Psychiatry, Bronx V.A. Medical Center, Bronx, New York and New York State University School of Medicine, New York, New York

Michael C. McLarnon, M.D.
Department of Psychiatry, Augusta V.A. Medical Center and Medical College of Georgia, Augusta, Georgia

Richard C. Mohs, Ph.D.
Department of Psychiatry, Bronx V.A. Medical Center, Bronx, New York and New York State University School of Medicine, New York, New York

Aron D. Mosnaim, Ph.D.
Department of Pharmacology, University of Health Sciences/The Chicago Medical School, North Chicago, Illinois

Henry A. Nasrallah, M.D.
Department of Psychiatry, Ohio State College of Medicine, Columbus, Ohio

Christine Nastase, M.D.
Douglas Hospital Centre and Department of Psychiatry, McGill University, Verdun, Quebec, Canada

Raymond Pass, Ph.D.
Department of Psychiatry, Columbia Presbyterian Medical Center, New York, New York

George N. Perelman, M.S.
Ida and Solomon Stern Psychiatry Research Unit, Beer Sheva Mental Health Center and Ben Gurion University of the Negev, Beer Sheva, Israel

Krishnaiah Rayasam, M.D.
Department of Psychiatry, Duke University Medical Center, Durham, North Carolina

Mary Ann Richardson, Ph.D.
Nathan S. Kline Institute for Psychiatric Research, Orangeburg, New York

Theresa A. Ryan, B.S.
Department of Psychiatry, Bronx V.A. Medical Center, Bronx, New York

Gabriel Schreiber, M.D., Ph.D.
Ida and Solomon Stern Psychiatry Research Unit, Beer Sheva Mental Health Center and Ben Gurion University of the Negev, Beer Sheva, Israel

George M. Simpson, M.D.
Department of Psychiatry, Medical College of Pennsylvania at Eastern Pennsylvania Psychiatric Institute, Philadelphia, Pennsylvania

Hardeep Singh, M.D.
Department of Psychiatry, Medical College of Pennsylvania at Eastern Pennsylvania Psychiatric Institute, Philadelphia, Pennsylvania

Robert C. Smith, M.D., Ph.D.
Department of Psychiatry, Albert Einstein College of Medicine, Bronx, New York

Stephen Michael Stahl, M.D., Ph.D.
University Department of Neurology, Institute of Psychiatry and Kings College Medical School, De Crespigny Park, London and Neuroscience Research Centre, Merck Sharp and Dohme Research Laboratories, Harlow, Essex, England

Carol A. Tamminga, M.D.
Maryland Psychiatric Research Center, University of Maryland, Baltimore, Maryland

Gunvant K. Thaker, M.D.
Maryland Psychiatric Research Center, University of Maryland, Baltimore, Maryland

Roberto Umansky, M.D.
Ida and Solomon Stern Psychiatry Research Unit, Beer Sheva Mental Health Center and Ben Gurion University of the Negev, Beer Sheva, Israel

Wim M. A. Verhoeven, M.D., Ph.D.
Department of Biological Psychiatry, Utrecht University Hospital, Utrecht, The Netherlands

John L. Waddington, M.A., Ph.D.
Department of Clinical Pharmacology, Royal College of Surgeons of Ireland, Dublin, Ireland

Marion E. Wolf, M.D.
Department of Psychiatry, North Chicago V.A. Medical Center, North Chicago and Loyola University, Stritch School of Medicine, Maywood, Illinois

Ramzy Yassa, M.D.
Department of Psychiatry, McGill University and Douglas Hospital Centre, Verdun, Quebec, Canada

Introduction to the
Progress in Psychiatry Series

T he *Progress in Psychiatry* Series is designed to capture in print the excitement that comes from assembling a diverse group of experts from various locations to examine in detail the newest information about a developing aspect of psychiatry. This series emerged as a collaboration between the American Psychiatric Association's Scientific Program Committee and the American Psychiatric Press, Inc. Great interest was generated by a number of the symposia presented each year at the APA Annual Meeting, and we realize that much of the information presented there, carefully assembled by people who are deeply immersed in a given area, would unfortunately not appear together in print. The symposia sessions at the Annual Meetings provide an unusual opportunity for experts who otherwise might not meet on the same platform to share their diverse viewpoints for a period of three hours. Some new themes are repeatedly reinforced and gain credence, while in other instances disagreements emerge, enabling the audience and now the reader to reach informed decisions about new directions in the field. The *Progress in Psychiatry* Series allows us to publish and capture some of the best of the symposia and thus provide an in-depth treatment of specific areas which might not otherwise be presented in broader review formats.

Psychiatry is by nature an interface discipline, combining the study of mind and brain, of individual and social environments, of the humane and the scientific. Therefore, progress in the field is rarely linear—it often comes from unexpected sources. Further, new developments emerge from an array of viewpoints that do not necessarily provide immediate agreement but rather expert examination of the issues. We intend to present innovative ideas and data that will enable you, the reader, to participate in this process.

We believe the *Progress in Psychiatry* Series will provide you with an opportunity to review timely new information in specific fields of interest as they are developing. We hope you find that the excitement of the presentations is captured in the written word and that this book proves to be informative and enjoyable reading.

David Spiegel, M.D.
Series Editor
Progress in Psychiatry Series

Introduction

This book was developed from the symposium "Tardive Dyskinesia: Biological Mechanisms and Clinical Aspects" held at
the annual meeting of the American Psychiatric Association, Chicago,
May 1987. It also incorporates manuscripts from other research
groups in an attempt to present an up-to-date, balanced view of
knowledge in this field.

In the first four chapters the various pathophysiological theories
of tardive dyskinesia, including the role of dopamine, acetylcholine,
gamma-aminobutyric acid (GABA), and neuroendocrine systems, are
examined. Chapter 5, on involuntary movements in the preneuroleptic era, gives a historical perspective. The classical clinical features
of the tardive dyskinesia syndrome are described in Chapter 6. The
important issues of long-term follow-up studies, comparison of patient characteristics associated with tardive dyskinesia versus those
associated with parkinsonism, tardive dyskinesia in the psychogeriatric population and in special populations, tardive dystonia, and
structural changes in the brain in this movement disorder are discussed in Chapters 7 through 12, respectively.

New therapeutic approaches in the management of tardive dyskinesia, such as the possible use of estrogens, GABA agents, and calcium
channel blockers, are discussed in Chapters 13 through 15, respectively. The study of the on–off dyskinesia syndrome of Parkinson's
disease may provide useful information for the understanding of the
phenomenology of tardive dyskinesia (Chapter 16). Chapter 17 is
devoted to novel antipsychotic compounds, whose possible efficacy
in the treatment of schizophrenia is studied with considerable interest,
given their decreased likelihood of extrapyramidal side effects. Another chapter examines the legal aspects of tardive dyskinesia and

presents the American Psychiatric Association's guidelines for the avoidance and management of tardive dyskinesia (Chapter 18). Finally, in Chapter 19, the focus shifts from the culprit drugs and predisposing conditions to the "human factor," as reflected in the resistance manifested by many mental health professionals to the implementation of measures aimed at the prevention and management of this disorder.

We wish to acknowledge the contributions of all authors to this book, and the encouragement given to us by Dr. Jochnan Wolf. This book is dedicated to the memory of Jochnan Wolf, M.D. (1911–1986) and Leon Wolf (1947–1986).

Marion E. Wolf, M.D.
Aron D. Mosnaim, Ph.D.

Chapter 1

Is the Dopaminergic Supersensitivity Theory of Tardive Dyskinesia Valid?

Robert C. Smith, M.D., Ph.D.

Chapter 1

Is the Dopaminergic Supersensitivity Theory of Tardive Dyskinesia Valid?

The dopaminergic supersensitivity theory of the pathophysiology of tardive dyskinesia (TD) has been the primary theory guiding much of the basic and clinical research and treatment of this disorder for the past 20 years. However, recent research raises questions as to the degree of empirical support this metapharmacological theory has received. Its validity and utility may need to be reconsidered. This chapter reviews the evidence for the dopaminergic supersensitivity theory of TD and briefly examines alternative neurotransmitter hypotheses that have recently been proposed.

In its purest form, this metapharmacological theory concentrates on the supersensitivity of postsynaptic dopamine receptors as they relate to the pathophysiology of TD. Key elements of this hypothesis include the following lines of reasoning: 1) Administration of neuroleptics blocks postsynaptic dopamine receptors in the striatum; 2) chronic blockade results in a supersensitivity of these dopamine receptors, similar to the denervation supersensitivity seen after surgical or chemical lesions; 3) supersensitivity in the striatal dopamine system leads to choreiform motor responses in many parts of the body; and 4) after long-term administration of neuroleptics this supersensitivity becomes relatively permanent, leading to the phenomenon of persistent TD. We shall review the evidence in terms of several predictions that can be derived from this theory.

PREDICTIONS AND EVIDENCE

Prediction 1. Chronic administration of neuroleptic drugs leads to a supersensitivity of postsynaptic dopamine receptors in the striatum.

There is considerable evidence from behaviorial and biochemical studies in several species of animals that chronic administration of neuroleptics produces a state of dopaminergic supersensitivity in the nigrostriatal system and possibly other parts of the brain. This has been consistently shown in behavioral pharmacological tests by increased stereotypy and gnawing response to dopamine agonists such as apomorphine and amphetamine (1–3). On a biochemical level it is evidenced by increased number of dopamine receptors, as indicated by radioligand binding studies (3–5), and altered dopamine metabolism or turnover after administration of dopamine agonists (4, 6) in the caudate or striatum.

Figure 1 shows an example from our own prior research of increased stereotyped behavior response to apomorphine during several weeks after cessation of drug treatment, in rats previously treated for three weeks with two doses of haloperidol. Figure 2 illustrates results of increased spiperone binding to dopamine receptors in the striatum after termination of chronic fluphenazine treatment. However, the behavioral supersensitivity peaks about one week after cessation of neuroleptics and is usually evident for only a few weeks after cessation of drug treatment. Increases in dopamine receptors are also a relatively short-lived phenomenon after termination of neuroleptic treatment to rats, and have been reported not to be present several months after termination of neuroleptics, when other behavioral manifestations of oral dyskinesia persist (7, 8).

Prediction 2. Drugs that block supposedly supersensitive dopamine receptors will decrease symptoms of TD. Drugs that decrease available dopamine to act on supersensitive dopamine receptors will decrease symptoms of TD.

There is considerable evidence that drugs that decrease dopaminergic transmission decrease symptoms of TD (9, 10). Increasing the dose of a neuroleptic, or restarting treatment with neuroleptic drugs, such as haloperidol, that block dopaminergic receptors, usually decreases motor symptoms of TD, although this effect is sometimes transitory, with dyskinesia symptoms breaking through and sometimes increasing after several weeks or months of treatment (11). It has been hypothesized that the breakthrough or aggravation of TD symptoms in this situation may be due to a continued expansion of neuroleptic receptors induced by the additional treatment, which cannot be blocked by the neuroleptic drug; it is also possible that modulation of dopamine receptors only affects the immediate expression of the motor symptoms and does not influence other aspects of the underlying pathophysiology.

Drugs that deplete dopamine, such as tetrabenazine, reserpine, and alpha-methylparatyrosine, have also been effective in reducing TD (12–14). The mechanism of this effect is probably due to the decrease

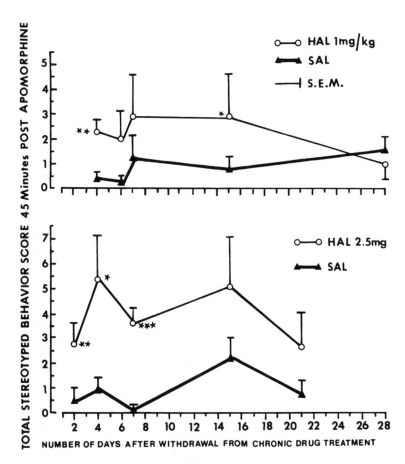

Figure 1. Stereotyped behavioral response to apomorphine in rats withdrawn from six to seven weeks of treatment with haloperidol (HAL) or saline (SAL), at indicated days after termination of chronic haloperidol. Each point represents mean total stereotyped behavior score on indicated day, 45 minutes after administration of 1 mg/kg apomorphine.

in brain dopamine available to activate the increased number of postsynaptic receptors. However, these therapeutic effects provide equal support to a hypothesis of presynaptic dopamine overactivity, rather than postsynaptic receptor supersensitivity.

Prediction 3. Administration of direct and indirect dopamine agonists should worsen symptoms of TD.

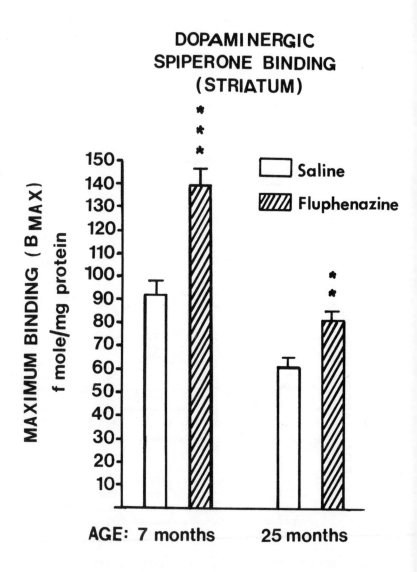

Figure 2. Increase in number of dopamine-2 receptors in rat caudate, indicated by increase in B_{max} of spiperone binding, in mature (7 months) and old (25 months) rats, sacrificed 10 days after termination of 2 months of treatment with fluphenazine hydrochloride (2 mg/kg) or saline.

Administration of putative drugs that directly stimulate postsynaptic dopamine receptors has shown that these drugs do not consistently increase the symptoms of tardive dyskinesia. In fact, the overall tendency is for reduction or no change in TD symptoms after acute or chronic administration of these drugs. Our own research (15), as well as that of others (16), shows overall reduction in TD symptoms in several patients after administration of apomorphine. Figure 3 presents results from our double-blind cross-over study in which we administered several doses of apomorphine and placebo to schizophrenic patients with TD. Several studies have also provided evidence that another dopamine agonist, bromocriptine, a drug that has direct stimulating effects on postsynaptic dopamine receptors as well as effects on presynaptic receptors and release, may ameliorate

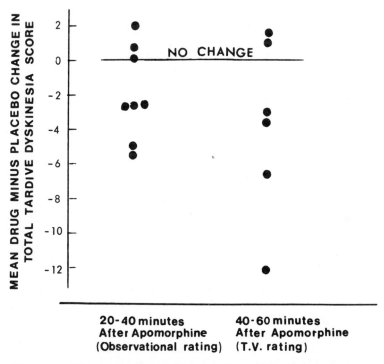

Figure 3. Effects of apomorphine on tardive dyskinesia scores in neuroleptic-free schizophrenic patients with tardive dyskinesia. Each point represents difference between mean scores on 2 to 5 active apomorphine days (doses 0.75 to 6.0 mg/kg subcutaneously) and 2 to 5 saline placebo days.

rather than exacerbate symptoms of TD. Results of these studies show that at both relatively high and low doses, bromocriptine generally diminishes symptoms of TD, with reduction of symptoms in a proportion of patients being greater than 50 percent (17–20).

Studies of the effects of indirect acting dopamine agonists, which release dopamine from the presynaptic neuron or increase precursor availability, have shown mixed results, although single acute doses of these drugs often transiently increase the symptoms of TD. Our own studies (15) have shown that administration of intravenous but not oral amphetamine to patients with TD temporarily increased ratings of TD symptoms at a time consistent with the drug's peak pharmacological effect. Administration of oral L-dopa or L-dopa/carbidopa for a short period of time has also been reported to increase dyskinesia scores in patients with TD (14, 21). However, chronic administration of L-dopa, in a titrated dose-increasing paradigm, has been reported to reduce symptoms of TD in up to 90 percent of patients studied in some series and with substantial reduction in TD symptom scores ($>$ 50 percent and up to 80 percent) (22, 23). This clinical effect has been proposed to be mediated by the gradual desensitization of dopamine receptors through increase in the agonist neurotransmitter dopamine. However, this therapeutic effect has not been confirmed by all investigators (24).

Prediction 4. Patients with TD will have a greater number of dopamine receptors in their striatum than patients without TD.

In the past few years receptor binding studies have been performed on postmortem specimens of brains of schizophrenic patients using radio-receptor binding techniques. Several reports have shown an increase in dopamine-2 (D-2) neuroleptic receptors (^{3}H-spiperone and ^{3}H-haloperidol binding) in the brains of schizophrenic patients compared to those of controls (25–28). In a small series comparing receptor binding in postmortem brain specimens of patients who exhibited or did not exhibit signs of TD before their death, there was no difference in either in the number or binding affinity of ligands to D-2 or D-1 receptors between patients with and without TD (29–30). This is contrary to expectations based on animal models discussed above and predictions stemming from a postsynaptic dopaminergic supersensitivity theory.

Prediction 5. Patients with TD should have lower homovanillic acid (HVA) levels than schizophrenic controls.

HVA is one of the main metabolites of dopamine and has been used as an indicator reflecting dopamine release or turnover. There is a feedback loop from the postsynaptic neuron to presynaptic neuron that modulates dopamine synthesis or release; it results in a decrease of available dopamine in response to increases in receptor stimulation, such as would occur in conditions leading to increased postsynaptic receptor number and/or overactivity of presynaptic dopamine neurons. Supersensitivity of postsynaptic dopamine receptors should lead to a compensatory decrease in dopamine release from the presynaptic neurons and, consequently, lower levels of HVA.

However, the experimental evidence on HVA levels in patients with TD is generally negative. In studies measuring cerebrospinal fluid (CSF) HVA in drug-free patients only one study has shown lower levels of HVA in patients with TD (31), while several other studies (32, 33) have reported no difference in CSF HVA between patients and controls, and one investigation reported higher levels of CSF HVA in patients with TD (34). One study of HVA levels in postmortem brain specimens reported higher levels of HVA in schizophrenic patients with TD than in schizophrenic patients without TD (29). Studies of TD patients during the period after withdrawal of neuroleptics have not yielded easily interpretable findings in regard to the supersensitivity hypothesis. Kirch et al. (35) reported a positive correlation between TD score and plasma HVA. Perenyi et al. (36) found less decrease in CSF HVA in schizophrenic patients with TD than in those without TD; this is not the result that would be expected on the basis of a dopaminergic supersensitivity hypothesis.

Prediction 6.   Patients with TD should have more pronounced changes in growth hormone and prolactin responses to dopamine agonists, such as apomorphine, or to dopamine antagonists, such as neuroleptics, than patients without TD.

Release of prolactin and growth hormone from the pituitary is mediated in important ways by dopaminergic influences in the tuberoinfundibular system, and numerous studies have shown that direct and indirect dopamine agonists such as apomorphine or L-dopa decrease plasma prolactin and increase plasma growth hormone in humans and animals. Dopamine antagonists such as neuroleptics increase plasma prolactin but do not have a marked effect on growth hormone. There is some evidence from studies in rats that the dopamine receptors in the tuberoinfundibular system may also become supersensitive after termination of chronic neuroleptic administration (37). If patients with TD had supersensitive postsynaptic dopamine receptors in the tuberoinfundibular system as well as the striatum, then we would expect patients with TD to show greater changes in prolactin and growth hormone response than schizophrenic patients without TD.

The experimental evidence appears to be conclusively negative on the prediction that patients with TD would have greater neuroendocrine responses to dopamine agonists or antagonists. Our own group (15, 38) has reported that (neuroleptic-free) patients with TD do not have a greater prolactin decrease or greater growth hormone increase after administration of subcutaneous apomorphine or oral L-dopa than do schizophrenic controls without TD. The most consistent finding was that chronic schizophrenic patients with or without TD had uniformly blunted neuroendocrine responses compared to normal controls in these dopaminergic neuroendocrine challenge tests. In contrast, some studies have found that acute schizophrenic patients have greater growth hormone responses to apomorphine than controls (39). Investigations of the prolactin response to challenge doses of neuroleptics have also shown that schizophrenic patients with TD do not have a greater increase in prolactin than schizophrenic patients without TD (40, 41).

Prediction 7. Schizophrenic patients with TD who are neuroleptic free should have low basal prolactin levels, and neuroleptic-treated schizophrenic patients should have higher basal prolactin levels than schizophrenic patients without TD.

Prediction 6 was based on the results of provocative challenge tests with dopaminergic drugs. Since dopamine is an inhibitory influence on prolactin secretion, we would also expect a patient with supersensitive dopamine receptors to have lower basal prolactin in the neuroleptic-free state and higher basal prolactin levels when treated with neuroleptics on a regular dosage schedule. This is based on the hypothesis that TD patients have an increased number of dopamine receptors that can be stimulated or blocked.

There are no published reports of basal prolactin levels in drug-free schizophrenic patients. The evidence on basal prolactin levels in neuroleptic-treated schizophrenic patients is contradictory. Tripodianakis et al. (42) reported no relationship between prolactin levels and the presence of TD. Glazer et al. (43) reported higher prolactin levels in neuroleptic-treated male TD patients but not female TD patients. Csernansky et al. (44) reported a significantly positive correlation between the severity of TD symptoms and the ratio of prolactin/serum neuroleptic levels in younger but not older TD patients. Brown and Laughren (45) reported increased basal secretion of growth hormone and a tendency for decreased basal prolactin secretion in schizophrenic patients terminated from neuroleptic drugs and showing withdrawal emergent dyskinesia, but no changes in these neuroendocrine parameters in patients with persistent TD.

Prediction 8. Prolonged treatment with neuroleptics should induce persistent symptoms of extrapyramidal motor disorder in animals that resemble symptoms of TD and that are correlated with indices of dopamine receptor supersensitivity.

More recent research in animal models does not support the conclusion that indices of dopaminergic supersensitivity found after treatment with neuroleptic drugs in animals are closely related to more relevant animal models of TD.

Although, as we have noted above (see prediction 1), chronic administration of neuroleptic drugs produces evidence of behavioral and biochemical dopaminergic supersensitivity, this supersensitivity is short lived. Even after a year of treatment with neuroleptic drugs, behavioral supersensitivity in rats persisted only 2 or 3 months (5).

In more recent research, spontaneous oral dyskinesia in the rat and monkey has been investigated as behavioral response that more closely resembles the primary features of TD in humans. This behavior increases during chronic administration of many neuroleptic drugs and persists for months after termination of neuroleptics. However, at a time when oral chewing persisted there was no evidence of increased brain dopamine receptors as assayed by receptor binding studies, and the extent of oral dyskinesia produced by neuroleptics was not correlated with the extent of increase in dopamine receptors produced by these drugs (7). Moreover, biochemical studies of the brains of monkeys who developed persistent TD after chronic administration of neuroleptics did not reveal differences in dopamine receptor bindings in the striatum of monkeys who developed persistent TD versus non-TD monkeys, but rather differences in enzymes related to the gamma-aminobutyric acid (GABA) synthesizing system of the brain (see below).

Summary

In summary, many of the predictions deriving from the dopaminergic supersensitivity hypothesis have not received consistent support. This has been detailed above and is summarized in Table 1. Although chronic administration of neuroleptic drugs increases dopamine receptors in rat brain, indices of dopamine supersensitivity have not been convincingly related to persistent dyskinesia in either patients or in animal models. There is some support for the idea of overactivity of presynaptic dopaminergic neurons from provocative drug tests in humans. The evidence reviewed is more in accord with the suggestion that dopaminergic supersensitivity may be more importantly involved in the withdrawal dyskinesia seen in some patients after termination of neuroleptics, which diminishes or completely vanishes within a relatively short time.

Table 1. Summary of evidence for predictions from postsynaptic dopaminergic supersensitivity theory of tardive dyskinesia (TD).

Prediction number	Hypothesis	State of the evidence	Implications for support of dopaminergic supersensitivity theory
1	Chronic neuroleptics produce dopaminergic supersensitivity	Consistently positive; confirmed	Supports theory
2a	Dopamine receptor antagonists reduce TD symptoms	Positive; confirmed some tolerance	Supports theory
2b	Presynaptic depleters reduce TD symptoms	Positive; confirmed	Supports theory, but equally supports other theories
3	Dopamine agonists increase TD symptoms		
3a	Direct receptor agonists	Negative; opposite effects	Theoretically important disconfirmation
3b	Indirect agonists, work through presynaptic neuron	Mixed; some positive evidence, some unexpected opposite effects	Supports theory, but equally consistent with other theories
4	Patients with TD have greater number of dopamine receptors in their brains	Negative; disconfirmation	Theoretically important disconfirmation

Table 1. (continued)

Prediction number	Hypothesis	State of the evidence	Implications for support of dopaminergic supersensitivity theory
5	TD patients have lower homovanillic acid than schizophrenic patients without TD	Mostly negative	Does not support theory; disconfirmation
6	TD patients will have greater neuroendocrine responses to dopamine agonists	Consistently negative	Does not support theory
7	Basal prolactin levels will be lower in drug-free and higher in neuroleptic-treated schizophrenic patients	Contradictory; mostly negative	Does not support theory
8	Dopaminergic supersensitivity will correlate with behavioral expression of TD-like symptoms in animal models	Recent evidence mostly negative	Does not support theory

ALTERNATIVE NEUROTRANSMITTERS

Recent research has suggested that other brain neurotransmitters, such as norepinephrine (NE) and GABA, may be pharmacologically more important in some of the pathophysiological mechanisms underlying TD and may provide alternatives to the dopamine supersensitivity hypothesis as the primary etiology of this syndrome.

Norepinephrine

Some of the evidence reviewed above that supposedly provided support for the dopaminergic supersensitivity hypotheses would also be consistent with hypotheses stemming from brain noradrenergic overactivity. Many neuroleptic drugs bind to brain adrenergic receptors as well as dopamine receptors. Chronic administration of neuroleptic drugs results in a supersensitivity of some brain adrenergic receptors on a behavioral (46) and biochemical (3) level. In fact, our previous research (4) with young and old rats has demonstrated an increase in the number of beta-adrenergic receptors in rat brain after termination of 2 months of fluphenazine treatment (see Figure 4). It is important to note that the increase in the B_{max} of beta-adrenergic receptors was much greater in the old-age rats than in the young adult rats; this would be consistent with the greater prevalence of TD in the older patient receiving neuroleptics. Messiha (47) has also reported increased urinary excretion of NE in monkeys who developed TD after chronic neuroleptic administration. Indirect dopamine agonists, such as amphetamine and L-dopa, which exacerbate TD symptoms in some patients, have pharmacological effects on presynaptic neurons that can lead to increased NE as well as increased dopamine in the synaptic cleft. Furthermore, drugs such as reserpine that decrease TD symptoms through presynaptic mechanisms, may decrease NE as well as dopamine. These pharmacological and animal studies provide a basis for examining the role of NE in clinical studies of TD.

Results of some clinical biochemical studies also support a more central role for NE in the pathophysiology of TD. One research group (48, 49) has shown that schizophrenic patients with TD have significantly higher levels of the enzyme dopamine β-hydroxylase (DBH), which converts dopamine to NE. Although this result was derived from measuring enzyme activity levels in the serum of patients, there may be a similar overactivity in brain DBH. This group also found a correlation between both (1) CSF levels of NE and (2) alpha-adrenergic receptor binding to platelets with the severity of TD; this is consistent with the hypothesis that increased NE and/or noradrenergic receptors is involved in the pathophysiology of TD.

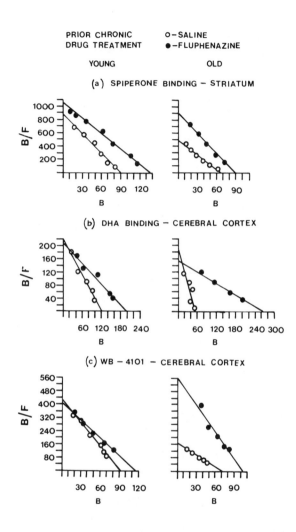

Figure 4. Greater effects of chronic fluphenazine on increasing beta-adrenergic receptors than dopaminergic receptors in old rats (25 months) terminated from chronic fluphenazine treatment. Figure illustrates representative schatchard plots for number of receptors (maximum binding) from radioligand binding experiments in caudate (dopaminergic binding) or cortex (adrenergic binding). Spiperone-antagonist ligand for D2 dopamine receptor; DHA = antagonist ligand for beta-adrenergic receptor; WB-4101 = antagonist ligand for alpha-adrenergic receptor.

One study, using a slightly different DBH assay (50) did not report increased serum DBH in patients with TD.

Several small-scale treatment studies have also shown some reduction in TD symptoms after open trials of clonidine, an alpha-adrenergic receptor agonist (51–53), or propranolol, a beta-adrenergic receptor blocking agent (54). Studies have also suggested that some, but not all, TD patients show amelioration of TD symptoms during treatment with inhibitors of the enzyme DBH such as fusaric acid (55).

GABA

Pharmacological evidence implicates GABA in the regulation of movement through the striatal-nigral pathway and extrapyramidal system (56–58). GABA functions as an inhibitory neurotransmitter in the striatal-nigral pathway, and high doses of GABA inhibit the effects of dopamine agonists such as apomorphine. With long-term neuroleptic treatment there are compensatory changes in the GABA system of the brain, including a decrease of GABA turnover and increase in the number of GABA receptors in the substantia nigra. Especially significant is the differential change in GABA synthesizing enzymes in Cebus appella monkeys who develop dyskinesia after chronic treatment with neuroleptics. Monkeys who developed TD had lower enzyme activity of glutamic acid decarboxylase in their globus pallidus and substantia nigra than monkeys who did not develop TD (59, 60). Consistent with the lower GABA levels and turnover described above in animal studies, a recent study has also shown that patients with TD had about 30 percent lower CSF GABA levels than schizophrenic patients without TD (57).

Clinical trials of GABA drugs have demonstrated their effectiveness in reducing symptoms of TD, although the clinical usefulness of many of these agents is limited by other side effects. Direct-acting GABA agonists, such as muscimol and progabide, have been shown to reduce symptoms of TD (58, 61–63). Several studies of drugs that inhibit enzymes mediating GABA destruction, for example, gamma-acetylenic GABA and gamma-vinyl GABA, also suggest that drugs that increase GABA levels decrease TD symptom scores (57, 64–66). Benzodiazepines, which appear to reduce symptoms of TD in a few open clinical trials or case reports, are putative GABA receptor enhancers (67).

Thus pharmacological, animal model, and clinical experimental trials all support a more central role for dysfunction in the brain GABA system as possibly more central in the underlying pathophysiology of the TD syndrome.

REFERENCES

1. Sayers AC, Burki HR, Ruch W, et al: Neuroleptic-induced hypersensitivity of striatal dopamine receptors in the rat as a model of tardive dyskinesia: effects of clozapine, haloperidol, loxapine, chlorpromazine. Psychopharmacology 41:97–104, 1975

2. Smith RC, Davis JM: Behavioral evidence for supersensitivity after chronic administration of haloperidol, clozapine, and thioridazine. Life Sci 19:725–732, 1976

3. Muller P, Seeman P: Dopaminergic supersensitivity after neuroleptics: time course and specificity. Psychopharmacology 60:1–11, 1978

4. Smith RC, Shelat HS, Sammeta J, et al: Aging, receptors, and neuroleptic drugs, in Brain Neurotransmitters and Receptors in Aging and Age Related Disorders. Edited by Enna SJ, Samorajshi T, Beer B. New York, Raven Press, 1981, pp. 231–243

5. Clow A, Theodorou A, Jenner P, et al: Central dopamine function in rats following withdrawal from one year of continuous neuroleptic administration. Eur J Pharmacol 63:145–157, 1980

6. Wheeler SC, Roth RH: Tolerance to fluphenazine and supersensitivity to apomorphine in central dopaminergic system after chronic fluphenazine decanoate treatment. Naunyn-Schmiedeberg's Archives of Pharmacology 312:151–159, 1980

7. Waddington JL, Cross AJ, Gambel SJ, et al: Spontaneous orofacial dyskinesia and dopaminergic function in rats after 6 months of neuroleptic treatment. Science 220:530–532, 1983

8. Baldessarini RJ, Cole JO, Davis JM, et al: Tardive Dyskinesia: A Task Force Report of the American Psychiatric Association. Washington, DC, American Psychiatric Association, 1980

9. Fog R: The effects of dopamine antagonists on spontaneous and tardive dyskinesia. Psychopharmacology Supplementum 2: Dyskinesia—Research and Treatment 118–121, 1985

10. Jeste DV, Wyatt RJ: Therapeutic strategies against tardive dyskinesia. Arch Gen Psychiatry 39:803–816, 1982

11. Kazamatsuri H, Chien C-P, Cole JO: Long-term treatment of tardive dyskinesia with haloperidol and tetrabenazine. Am J Psychiatry 130:479–483, 1973

12. Fahn S: Long-term treatment of tardive dyskinesia with presynaptically acting dopamine-depleting agents, in Experimental Therapeutics of Movement Disorders. Edited by Fahn S, Calne DB, Shoulson I. New York, Raven Press, 1983, pp. 267–276

13. Fahn S: A therapeutic approach to tardive dyskinesia. J Clin Psychiatry 46[4, Sec 2]:19–24, 1985

14. Gerlach J, Reisby N, Randrup A: Dopaminergic hypersensitivity and cholinergic hypofunction in the pathophysiology of tardive dyskinesia. Psychopharmacologia 34:21–35, 1974

15. Smith RC, Tamminga CA, Haraszti J, et al: Effects of dopamine agonists in tardive dyskinesia. Am J Psychiatry 134:763–768, 1977

16. Carroll BJ, Curtis GC, Kokmen E: Paradoxical response to dopamine agonists in tardive dyskinesia. Am J Psychiatry 134:785–788, 1977

17. Lenox RH, Weaver LA, Saran BM: Tardive dyskinesia clinical and neuroendocrine response to low dose bromocriptine. J Clin Psychopharmacol 5:286–292, 1985

18. Tamminga CA, Chase TN: Bromocriptine and CF-397 in the treatment of tardive dyskinesia. Arch Neurol 37:204–205, 1980

19. Haggstrom J-E, Andersson U, Gunne LM: Bromocriptine in tardive dyskinesia. Pharmacopsychiatria 15:161–163, 1982

20. Jeste DV, Cutler NR, Kaufmann CA, et al: Low-dose apomorphine and bromocriptine in neuroleptic-induced movement disorders. Biol Psychiatry 18:1085–1091, 1983

21. Klawans HL, McKenall RR: Observations on the effect of levodopa on tardive lingual–facial–buccal dyskinesia. J Neurol Sci 14:189–192, 1971

22. Alpert M, Friedhoff AJ, Diamond F: Use of dopamine receptor agonists to reduce dopamine receptor number as treatment for tardive dyskinesia, in Advances in Neurology: Vol. 37. Experimental Therapeutics of Movement Disorders. Edited by Fahn S, Calne DB, Shoulson I. New York, Raven Press, 1983, pp. 253–258

23. Shoulson I: Carbidopa/levodopa therapy of coexistent drug-induced parkinsonism and tardive dyskinesia, in Advances in Neurology: Vol. 37. Experimental Therapeutics of Movement Disorders. Edited by Fahn S, Calne DB, Shoulson I. New York, Raven Press, 1983, pp. 259–266

24. Casey DE, Gerlach J, Bjoundal N: Levodopa and receptor sensitivity modification in tardive dyskinesia. Psychopharmacology 78:89–92, 1982

25. Lee T, Seeman P: Elevation of brain neuroleptic/dopamine receptors in schizophrenia: Am J Psychiatry 137:191–197, 1980

26. Seeman P: Brain dopamine receptors in schizophrenia and tardive dyskinesia. Psychopharmacology Supplementum 2: Dyskinesia—Research and Treatment 2–8, 1985

27. Owen F, Cross AJ, Crow TJ, et al: Increased dopamine receptor sensitivity in schizophrenia. Lancet 2:223–225, 1978

28. Cross AJ, Crow TJ, Owen F: H-flupenthixol binding in the brains of schizophrenics: evidence for a selective increase in D2 receptors. Psychopharmacology 74:122–124, 1981

29. Cross AJ, Crow TJ, Ferrier IN, et al: Chemical and structural changes in the brain in patients with movement disorders. Psychopharmacology Supplementum 2: Dyskinesia—Research and Treatment 104–110, 1985

30. Crow TJ, Cross AJ, Johnstone EC, et al: Abnormal involuntary movements in schizophrenia: are they related to the disease process or its treatment? Are they associated with changes in dopamine receptors? J Clin Psychopharmacol 82:336–340, 1982

31. Chase TN: Catecholamine metabolism in neurologic disease, in Frontiers in Catecholamine Research. Edited by Usdin E, Snyder S. New York, Pergamon Press, 1983, pp. 1127–1132

32. Bowers MB, Moore D, Tarsy D: Tardive dyskinesia: a clinical test of the supersensitivity hypothesis. Psychopharmacology 61:137–141, 1979

33. Nagao T, Ohsimo T, Mitsunobu K: Cerebrospinal fluid monoamine metabolites and cyclic nucleotides in chronic schizophrenic patients with tardive dyskinesia or drug-induced tremor. Biol Psychiatry 14:509–523, 1979

34. Pind K, Faurbye A: Concentration of HVA and 5-HIAA in the CSF after treatment with probenecid in patients with drug-induced tardive dyskinesia. Acta Psychiatr Scand 46:323–326, 1970

35. Kirch D, Hattox S, Bell C, et al: Plasma homovanillic acid and tardive dyskinesia during neuroleptic maintenance and withdrawal. Psychiatry Res 9:217–233, 1983

36. Perenyi A, Frecska E, Bagdy G, et al: Changes in mental condition, hyperkinesis and biochemical parameters after withdrawal of chronic neuroleptic treatment. Acta Psychiatr Scand 72:430–435, 1985

37. Lal H, Brown W, Drawbaugh R, et al: Enhanced prolactin inhibition following chronic treatment with haloperidol and morphine. Life Sci 20:101–106, 1977

38. Tamminga CA, Smith RC, Pandey G, et al: A neuroendocrine study of supersensitivity in tardive dyskinesia. Arch Gen Psychiatry 34:1199–1203, 1977

39. Pandey GN, Garver DL, Tamminga CA, et al: Post-synaptic supersensitivity in schizophrenia. Am J Psychiatry 134:518–522, 1977

40. Asnis G, Sachar E, Langer G, et al: Normal prolactin responses in tardive dyskinesia. Psychopharmacology 66:247–250, 1979

41. Wolf ME, Bowie L, Keener S, et al: Prolactin response in tardive dyskinesia. Biol Psychiatry 17:485–490, 1982

42. Tripodianakis J, Markianos M, Garelis E: Neurochemical studies of tardive dyskinesia I. Urinary homovanillic acid and plasma prolactin. Biol Psychiatry 18:337–345, 1983

43. Glazer WM, Moore DC, Bowers MB, et al: Serum prolactin and tardive dyskinesia. Am J Psychiatry 138:1493–1496, 1981

44. Csernansky JG, Prosser E, Kaplan J, et al: Possible associations among plasma prolactin levels, tardive dyskinesia, and paranoia in treated male schizophrenics. Biol Psychiatry 21:632–642, 1986

45. Brown WA, Laughren TP: Growth-hormone release and the tardive dyskinesia of neuroleptic withdrawal. Lancet 1:259, 1980

46. Dustan R, Jackson DM: The demonstration of a change in adrenergic receptor sensitivity in the central nervous system of mice after withdrawal from long-term treatment with haloperidol. Psychopharmacology 48:105–114, 1976

47. Messiha FJ: Biochemical studies after chronic administration of neuroleptics to monkeys, in Tardive Dyskinesia: Research and Treatment. Edited by Fann WE, Smith RC, Davis JM, et al. New York, Spectrum Publications, 1980

48. Jeste DV, DeLisi LE, Zalcman S, et al: A biochemical study of tardive dyskinesia in young male patients. Psychiatry Res 4:327–331, 1981

49. Kaufmann CA, Jeste DV, Shelton RC, et al: Noradrenergic and neuroradiological abnormalities in tardive dyskinesia. Biol Psychiatry 21:799–812, 1986

50. Markianos M, Tripodianakis J, Garelis E: Neurochemical studies of tardive dyskinesia II. Urinary methoxyhydroxyphenylglycol and plasma dopamine-B-hydroxylase. Biol Psychiatry 3:347–354, 1983

51. Freedman R, Kirch DG, Adler M: Clonidine treatment of schizophrenia: double-blind comparison to placebo and neuroleptic drugs. Acta Psychiatr Scand 65:25–45, 1982

52. Tripodianakis J, Markianos M: Clonidine trial in tardive dyskinesia, therapeutic response, MHPG, and plasma DBH. Pharmacopsychiatry 19:365–367, 1986

53. Browne J, Silver H, Martin R, et al: The use of clonidine in the treatment of neuroleptic-induced tardive dyskinesia. J Clin Psychopharmacol 6:88–92, 1986

54. Bacher NM, Lewis HA: Low-dose propranolol in tardive dyskinesia. Am J Psychiatry 137:495–497, 1980

55. Viukari M, Linnoila M: Effect of fusaric acid on tardive dyskinesia and mental state in psychogeriatric patients. Acta Psychiatr Scand 56:57–61, 1977

56. Scatton B, Gage D, Oblin A, et al: Influence of GABA mimetics and lithium on biochemical manifestation of striatal dopamine target cell hypersensitivity. Psychopharmacology Supplementum 2: Dyskinesia—Research and Treatment 29–44, 1985

57. Thaker GK, Tamminga CA, Alps LD, et al: Brain gamma-aminobutyric acid abnormality in tardive dyskinesia. Arch Gen Psychiatry 44:522–529, 1987

58. Tamminga CA, Thaker GK, Chase TN: GABA dysfunction in the pathophysiology of tardive dyskinesia. Psychopharmacology Supplementum 2: Dyskinesia—Research and Treatment 112–126, 1985

59. Gunne L-M, Haggstrom J-E: Reduction of nigral glutamic acid decarboxylase in rats with neuroleptic induced oral dyskinesia. Psychopharmacology 81:191–194, 1983

60. Gunne L-M, Haggstrom J-E, Sjoquist B: Association with persistent neuroleptic-induced dyskinesia of regional changes in brain GABA synthesis. Nature 309:347–349, 1984

61. Tamminga CA, Crayton JW, Chase TN: Improvement in tardive dyskinesia after muscimol therapy. Arch Gen Psychiatry 36:595–598, 1979

62. Korsgaard S, Casey DE, Gerlach J: Effect of gamma-vinyl GABA in tardive dyskinesia. Psychiatry Res 8:261–269, 1983

63. Morselli PL, Fournier V, Bossi L, et al: Clinical activity of GABA agonists in neuroleptic- and L-dopa-induced dyskinesia. Psychopharmacology Supplementum 2: Dyskinesia—Research and Treatment 128–135, 1985

64. Casey D, Gerlach J, Magelund G, et al: Gamma-acetylenic GABA in tardive dyskinesia. Arch Gen Psychiatry 37:1376–1379, 1980

65. Tell GP, Schecter PJ, Koch-Weser J, et al: Effects of gamma-vinyl GABA. N Engl J Med 305:581–582, 1981

66. Stahl SM, Thorton JE, Simpson ML, et al: Gamma-vinyl GABA treatment of tardive dyskinesia and other movement disorders. Biol Psychiatry 20:888–893, 1985

67. Bobruff A, Gardos G, Tarsy D, et al: Clonazepam and phenobarbital in tardive dyskinesia. Am J Psychiatry 138:189–193, 1981

Chapter 2

Implications of Muscarinic Receptor Heterogeneity for Research on Tardive Dyskinesia

Gabriel Schreiber, M.D., Ph.D.
Sofia Avissar, Ph.D.
Roberto Umansky, M.D.
George N. Perelman, M.S.
Robert H. Belmaker, M.D., Ph.D.

Chapter 2

Implications of Muscarinic Receptor Heterogeneity for Research on Tardive Dyskinesia

Anticholinergic drugs are useful in alleviating symptoms of parkinsonism, but these drugs exacerbate the abnormal movements of tardive dyskinesia. Some authors have claimed that prolonged exposure to anticholinergic drugs increases the risk of neuroleptic-induced tardive dyskinesia.

Substantial evidence has accumulated in recent years supporting the classification of muscarinic receptors into different subtypes, differentiated by drugs such as pirenzepine, which affect each subclass selectively (1–4). Muscarinic receptors in the cortex, hippocampus, striatum, and glandular tissues are designated type 1 (M-1, of high affinity to pirenzepine), while receptors in the heart and in intestinal smooth muscle are designated type 2 (M-2, of low affinity to pirenzepine). Radiographic studies in human and animal brain, using several selective and nonselective muscarinic antagonists, confirm different anatomic localization of M-1 and M-2 sites in brain (5, 6).

It is usually assumed that no biochemical or pharmacological differences exist among the various anticholinergic drugs used to relieve extrapyramidal side effects in psychiatric patients treated with neuroleptic drugs (7). The selection of anticholinergic drugs has been a matter of arbitrary choice. The recent discovery of subclasses of muscarinic receptors makes possible a definition of the pattern of muscarinic selectivity of each of the commonly used antiparkinsonian–anticholinergic drugs and raises the possibility that specific anticholinergic drugs might relieve parkinsonism without increasing risk of tardive dyskinesia.

We recently studied the interaction of the commonly used antiparkinsonian–anticholinergic drugs (biperiden, procyclidine, trihexyphenidyl, benztropine, methixen) with the muscarinic cholinergic receptor in a variety of rat tissues. The extent of the binding of each drug to the receptor was determined by measuring inhibition of the receptor-specific binding of [^{3}H]QNB.

Inhibition–concentration curves for the binding of these drugs in tissue preparations from cerebellum and ventricles (predominantly populated by M-2 receptors) and cortex, striatum, and hippocampus (predominantly populated by M-1 receptors) were prepared. The differences between the binding patterns of these drugs are striking. Methixen shows no selectivity in binding to any of the tissues studied. It may be defined as a nonselective muscarinic antagonist. In contrast, biperiden displays an approximately 15 times greater affinity for tissues populated with M-1 receptors than for the other tissues. Biperiden is, therefore, defined as an M-1 selective muscarinic antagonist with binding selectivity similar to pirenzepine. The other anticholinergic drugs show a range of selectivity. Benztropine, trihexyphenidyl, and procyclidine had, respectively, 2, 5, and 10 times higher affinities toward M-1 receptor-populated tissues. These data are summarized in Table 1.

Since M-1 muscarinic receptors predominate in the striatum, which is the target region of antiparkinsonian–anticholinergic medication, the finding of M-1 selective drugs among the anticholinergics makes such drugs a suitable first clinical choice in dystonia or parkinsonism. The advantage of treatment with M-1 selective drugs would be an expected sparsity of peripheral antimuscarinic side effects, since the majority of peripheral muscarinic receptors are of type 2.

However, the central nervous system contains muscarinic receptors of both M-1 and M-2 subtypes. Separate functions for these receptor subtypes have not yet been defined. However, preliminary results in our laboratory (Umansky, unpublished data, 1987) suggest that nonselective blockers reverse reserpine-induced hypomotility in mice, whereas M-1 receptor blockers do not. We are presently conducting experiments using apomorphine-induced stereotype as a model for tardive dyskinesia (8, 9), comparing chronic treatment with haloperidol alone, chronic treatment with haloperidol plus methixen, chronic treatment with haloperidol plus biperiden, and chronic treatment with haloperidol plus trihexyphenidyl. After 3 weeks of haloperidol treatment, with or without anticholinergic addition, treatments are stopped and apomorphine-induced stereotypy is evaluated after a 48-hour washout. We hypothesize that differences may exist between anticholinergic drugs in the tendency to increase haloperidol-induced supersensitivity of dopaminergic behavior. Such data from animal models may be relevant in planning human studies to reduce the risk of tardive dyskinesia inherent in treatment with neuroleptics plus anticholinergics.

Table 1. Comparison between affinities of various antiparkinsonian–anticholinergic drugs to the two subtypes of muscarinic receptors.

Receptor	Methixen		Benztropine		Trihexyphenidyl		Procyclidine		Biperiden	
	IC_{50cor} [a] (nM)	Relative affinity [b]	IC_{50cor} (nM)	Relative affinity	IC_{50cor} (nM)	Relative affinity	IC_{50cor} (nM)	Relative affinity	IC_{50cor} (nM)	Relative affinity
M-1 tissues										
Cortex	16.0	1.1	5.0	2.6	9.4	4.7	12.0	7.8	2.7	14.0
Hippocampus	16.0	1.1	5.0	2.6	10.1	4.0	15.0	6.3	3.8	10.0
Striatum	16.5	1.0	6.6	2.0	12.0	3.7	16.0	5.9	4.4	9.5
M-2 tissues										
Cerebellum	17.0	1.0	12.0	1.1	39.0	1.1	94.0	1.0	38.0	1.0
Ventricle	17.0	1.0	13.0	1.0	44.0	1.0	94.0	1.0	38.0	1.0

[a] Concentration of the drug causing 50 percent reduction in binding of $[^3H]$ QNB. IC_{50cor} values were calculated as $IC_{50cor} = IC_{50}/(1 + [C]/K_D)$, where K_D and (C) represent the dissociation constant and the concentration of $[^3H]$ QNB, respectively. K_D values for the binding of $[^3H]$ QNB to cortex, hippocampus, striatum, cerebellum, and ventricle were 0.25, 0.23, 0.22 and 0.20 nM, respectively.

[b] Value for the ventricle divided by IC_{50cor} value for the specified tissue.

REFERENCES

1. Gil DW, Wolff BB: Pirenzepine distinguishes between muscarinic receptor-mediated phosphoinositide breakdown and inhibition of adenylate cyclase. J Pharmacol Exp Ther 232:608–616, 1985

2. Hammer R, Berrie CP, Birdsall NJM, et al: Pirenzepine distinguishes between different subclasses of muscarinic receptors. Nature 283:90–92, 1980

3. Hammer R, Giachetti A: Muscarinic receptor subtypes: M1 and M2, biochemical and functional characterization. Life Sci 31:2991–2998, 1982

4. Watson M, Roeske WR, Yamamura HI: [³H] Pirenzepine selectively identifies a high affinity population of muscarinic cholinergic receptors in the rat cerebral cortex. Life Sci 31:2019–2023, 1982.

5. Cortes R, Palacios JM: Muscarinic cholinergic receptor subtypes in the rat brain: quantitative autoradiographic studies. Brain Res 362:227–238, 1986

6. Cortes R, Probst A, Tobler HJ, et al: Muscarinic cholinergic receptor subtypes in human brain: quantitative autoradiographic studies. Brain Res 362:239–253, 1986

7. Bianchine JR: Drugs for Parkinson's disease, in The Pharmacological Basis of Therapeutics. Edited by Gilman LS, Gilman A. New York, Macmillan, 1980, pp 475–493.

8. Bannet J, Belmaker RH, Ebstein RP: Clinical implications of the molecular model of tardive dyskinesia, in Neurotransmitters and Their Receptors. Edited by Littauer UZ, Dudai Y, Silman I, Teichberg VI, Vogel Z. New York, John Wiley, 1980, pp. 155–162

9. Globus M, Bannet J, Lerer B, et al: The effect of chronic bromocriptine and L-dopa on spiperone binding and apomorphine-induced stereotypy. Psychopharmacology 78:81–84, 1982

Chapter 3

The GABA Theory of Tardive Dyskinesia

Lars M. Gunne, M.D.
Edward D. Levin, Ph.D.
Per E. Johansson, M.D.

Chapter 3

The GABA Theory of Tardive Dyskinesia

In recent years a variety of studies have provided evidence that alterations in gamma-aminobutyric acid (GABA) function may underlie the increases in oral activity seen in tardive dyskinesia (TD). Support for this theory comes from both behavioral and neurochemical studies in humans with tardive dyskinesia and animal models of this syndrome.

It is commonly accepted that TD results from chronic administration of dopamine (DA) receptor blockers, although it is well known that oral dyskinesias, indistinguishable from TD, may occur in elderly patients who have received no neuroleptic treatment (1, 2). The relationship between DA receptor blockade and TD is further clouded by the fact that schizophrenic-related stereotypies, which may resemble TD, were known to occur before the advent of neuroleptic treatment (3). Most research into the neural dysfunction underlying TD has focused on the striatum and substantia nigra, because these are classic motor areas and because the nigrostriatal track contains one of the largest DA projections in the brain. The most prominent theory of the neural basis of TD is the DA supersensitivity hypothesis, which states that the increase in movement seen in TD results from the increase in DA receptor sensitivity caused by chronic DA receptor blockade. One of the problems with this theory is the timing of DA receptor supersensitivity. It can be seen even when the period of neuroleptic administration is short and has even been seen after a single injection of haloperidol (4, 5). In contrast, TD takes many months or years to develop. This difference in timing is also seen after withdrawal from neuroleptic drug administration. DA receptor supersensitivity rather quickly disappears, while TD persists for a much longer time and is often permanent.

This work was supported by the Swedish MRC grant no. 4546.

Another major problem with the DA receptor supersensitivity theory of TD concerns the selectivity of the effect. DA receptor supersensitivity affects all individuals given chronic neuroleptic treatment, whereas only some individuals develop TD. Our investigations with rats and monkeys have found that chronic neuroleptic administration causes persistent changes in the GABA system that selectively occur in the individuals showing dyskinesia or increases in oral activity.

GABA neurons provide several key points of control in the nigrostriatal loop. GABA interneurons are abundant in both the striatum and the substantia nigra, and GABA projection neurons form a major link from the striatum to the substantia nigra. The GABA neurons in the nigrostriatal loop have been found to be involved in motor behavior (6–9). In particular, this is true for oral movement. GABA neurons in the striatum and substantia nigra have been found to mediate the effects of DA drugs on oral behavior (10). Subchronic administration of neuroleptic drugs leads to supersensitivity to the effects of intranigral infusion of the GABA agonists, muscimol, tetrahydroisozolopyridinol (THIP), and baclofen (11, 12). It also has been found to reduce nigral GABA turnover rate (13); reduce the activity of glutamic acid decarboxylase (GAD), the GABA synthetic enzyme (14); and increase GABA binding in the substantia nigra (15). It is reasonable to expect that alterations in the effect of nigrostriatal DA neurons caused by long-term neuroleptic administration would also have effects on GABA neurons in the nigrostriatal-nigral loop. Studies in our laboratory further support the importance of GABA in the dyskinetic effects of long-term neuroleptic treatment.

STUDIES IN OUR LABORATORY

Of particular interest in our laboratory is the relationship of the reduction in GAD activity with the increase in dyskinetic activity in rats and Cebus apella monkeys chronically administered neuroleptics. These studies have found that the reduction in GAD activity fulfills two of the major shortcomings of the DA supersensitivity theory of TD: It is persistent after neuroleptic withdrawal, and it occurs only in those individuals who show neuroleptic-induced dyskinesia.

In experiments with both rats and Cebus monkeys we have found that the neuroleptic-induced dyskinesia is delayed in onset and persists for a prolonged period after withdrawal. In a study with rats (16) we found that monthly injections with haloperidol decanoate did not produce increases in vacuous chewing movements until 4 months after the onset of administration. This effect persisted for the remainder of the period of drug administration and for at least 4 months after withdrawal. At this time GAD activity in the substantia nigra was found to be markedly decreased in the neuroleptic treated rats. With Cebus monkeys it has taken between 3 months and 3 years of neuroleptic drug administration to induce a dyskinetic syndrome (17). After withdrawal, the dyskinesia has persisted for at least 1 year and in one case has lasted for up to 8 years (18). Two months after withdrawal of neuroleptic administration a subset of the monkeys was sacrificed for GAD analysis. As with the rats, significant decreases in GAD activity were seen in the substantia nigra. In addition, significant decreases were also seen in the subthalamic nucleus and medial globus pallidus (19).

DISCUSSION

From clinical studies there are a variety of findings that may support the GABA theory of TD. Decreased GABA levels in the cerebrospinal fluid have been found in schizophrenic patients with TD compared to those without TD (20). As has been seen in rats studies (21, 22), drug treatments that increase the stimulation of GABA receptors or increase GABAergic transmission have been found to ameliorate the symptoms of TD. Several studies have found that inhibition of the GABA degradative enzyme, GABA-transaminase, alleviates the dyskinesia associated with TD (20, 23–27). GABA agonists have been found to be effective in attenuating the motor symptoms of TD (28). The directly acting GABA agonists—muscimol (29), THIP (20), progabide (30)—all have been found to improve TD. Singh et al. (31) found that diazepam, which increases the effect of GABA, is also useful in treating TD. However, other investigators have not found GABA agonists to be effective in treating TD (32). The GABA receptor agonist baclofen has been tried by several groups without success in alleviating TD symptoms (33–36). Another agonist, sodium valproate, has also been tried without success (37, 38). One problem with the use of GABA agonists in the treatment of TD is the ubiquity of GABA in the brain. One cannot expect that systemic administration of the GABA agonist would enhance GABA effects only in the substantia nigra and the enhancement of GABA action in other motor areas may have quite different effects. Despite this nonspecificity, Thaker et al. (20) suggest that the decrease in cerebrospinal fluid GABA and the degree to which some GABA agonists do have beneficial effects support the importance of nigral GABA neurons in suppressing dyskinetic movements (20).

The data supporting the involvement of GABA with TD that we and others have collected are fairly convincing, especially in terms of the timing of the effect and individual differences in susceptibility, but some investigators have not found significant decreases in nigral

GAD activity after chronic neuroleptic administration (22, 39, 40). Lloyd and Hornykiewicz (39) administered haloperidol (20 mg/kg/ day) to rats for 24 weeks. They did not find a significant decrease in nigral GAD activity, although there was a trend in that direction. The haloperidol-treated rats had an average of 85.4 percent of the activity of the controls. Given the fact that there were only five rats in the haloperidol group, the lack of statistical significance in their study may be related to inadequate statistical power. In a larger study, Mithani et al. (22) gave haloperidol decanoate (28.5 mg/kg every 3 weeks) on the same schedule as Gunne and Haggstrom (16). Support for the GABA theory in this study was mixed. In favor of this theory, they found a significant decrease in nigral GAD after 40 weeks of haloperidol administration and found that the haloperidol-induced increase in vacuous chewing movements was attenuated by the GABA agonist progabide. On the other hand, they did not find any significant changes in nigral GAD activity after 16 or 48 weeks of exposure or 16 weeks after withdrawal. It is unclear why the decrease in GAD activity seen at 40 weeks was not also seen after 8 additional weeks of exposure. Our experience with both the primate and the rodent model has necessarily delivered only fragmentary knowledge of when and under what circumstances GABA mechanisms are altered during chronic neuroleptic treatment and withdrawal. Obviously oral and other dyskinetic movements appear long before there are measurable depressions of nigral GAD activity (provided GAD activity is measured after the addition of the cofactor pyridoxal phosphate). When cofactor was not added, Itoh (14) found reductions in nigral GAD activity after only 2 weeks of neuroleptic administration, that is, a time point when oral dyskinesias have not yet emerged. In our opinion the reductions of cofactor-saturated GAD activity noticed in our work should be ascribed to a loss of striatonigral GABA neuron terminals, representing an end point in a development involving longstanding striatonigral GABA neuron inhibition. Low nigral GAD activity may thus be a marker of irreversible brain damage. In support of this view, we have seen these GABA and GAD depressions only in monkeys with irreversible dyskinesias and in rats after experiments of more than a year's duration.

Support for the GABA theory of TD comes from a variety of sources, both experimental and clinical. A major point in favor of this theory is the finding that the GABA systems of some individuals are affected by chronic neuroleptic administration while others are not. However, this also presents problems in the development of animal models to test this theory. The same factors that alter individual sensitivity can also alter the sensitivity of whole groups of animals in a particular study. It is then important to discover the factors critical in determining the sensitivity of the GABA system to the effects of chronic neuroleptic administration. This will not only facilitate the conduct of reproducible studies but also may lead to a greater understanding of the mechanisms behind the individual differences in susceptibility to TD.

REFERENCES

1. Kane JM, Smith JM: Tardive dyskinesia: prevalence and risk factors, 1959 to 1979. Arch Gen Psychiatry 39:473–481, 1982

2. Kane JM, Weinhold P, Kinon B, et al: Prevalence of abnormal involuntary movements ("spontaneous dyskinesias") in the normal elderly. Psychopharmacology 77:105–108, 1982

3. Marsden CD: Is tardive dyskinesia a unique disorder? Psychopharmacology Supplementum 2: Dyskinesia—Research and Treatment 64–71, 1985

4. Asper H, Baggiolini M, Burki HR, et al: Tolerance phenomena with neuroleptics catalepsy, apomorphine stereotypies and striatal dopamine metabolism in the rat after single and repeated administration of loxapine and haloperidol. Eur J Pharmacol 22:287–294, 1973

5. Christenson AV, Fjalland B, Nielsen IM: On the supersensitivity of dopamine receptors induced by neuroleptics. Psychopharmacol 48: 1–6, 1976

6. Chase TM, Tamminga CA: GABA system participation in motor, cognitive and endocrine function in man, in GABA-Neurotransmitters: Pharmacochemical, Biochemical and Pharmacological Aspects. Edited by Korsgaard-Larsen P, Scheel-Kruger J, Kofod H. New York, Academic Press, 1979, pp 283–296

7. Gale K, Casu M: Dynamic utilization of GABA substantia nigra: regulation by dopamine and GABA in the striatum and its clinical and behavioral implications. Mol Cell Biochem 39:369–405, 1981

8. Scheel-Kruger J: The GABA receptor and animal behaviour evidence that GABA transmits and mediates dopaminergic functions in the basal ganglia and the limbic system, in GABA Receptors. Edited by Enna SJ. Clifton, NJ, Humana Press, 1983, pp. 215–255

9. Scheel-Kruger J, Magelund G, Olinas MC: Role of GABA in the striatal output system: globus pallidus, nucleus entopeduncularis, substantia

nigra and nucleus subthalamicus, in GABA and the Basal Ganglia. Edited by DiChiara G, Gessa GL. New York, Raven Press, 1981, pp. 165–186

10. Scheel-Kruger J, Arnt J: New aspects of the role of dopamine, acetylcholine and GABA in the development of tardive dyskinesia. Psychopharmacology Supplementum 2: Dyskinesia—Research and Treatment 46–71, 1985

11. Coward DM: Classical and non-classical neuroleptics induce supersensitivity of nigral GABAergic mechanisms in the rat. Psychopharmacology 78:180–184, 1982

12. Coward DM: Nigral actions of GABA agonists are enhanced by chronic fluphenazine and differentiated by concomitant flurazepam. Psychopharmacology 76:294–298, 1982

13. Mao CC, Cheney DL, Marco E, et al: Turnover times of gamma-aminobutyric acid and acetylcholine in nucleus caudatus, nucleus accumbens, globus pallidus and substantia nigra: effects of repeated administration of haloperidol. Brain Res 132:375–379, 1977

14. Itoh M: Effect of haloperidol on glutamate decarboxylase activity in discrete brain areas in the rat. Psychopharmacology 79:169–172, 1983

15. Gale K: Chronic blockade of dopamine receptors by antischizophrenic drugs enhances GABA binding in the substantia nigra. Nature 283:569–570, 1980

16. Gunne LM, Haggstrom JE: Reduction of nigral glutamic acid decarboxylase in rats with neuroleptic-induced oral dyskinesia. Psychopharmacology 81:191–194, 1983

17. Barany S, Ingvast A, Gunne LM: Development of acute dystonia and tardive dyskinesia in Cebus monkeys. Res Commun Chem Pathol Pharmacol 25:269–279, 1979

18. Gunne LM, Barany S: A monitoring test for the liability of neuroleptic drugs to induce tardive dyskinesia. Psychopharmacology 63:195–198, 1979

19. Gunne LM, Haggstrom JE, Sjoquist B: Association with persistent neuroleptic-induced dyskinesia of regional changes in brain GABA synthesis. Nature 309:347–349, 1984

20. Thaker GK, Tamminga CA, Alphs LD, et al: Brain gamma-aminobutyric acid abnormality in tardive dyskinesia. Arch Gen Psychiatry 44:522–529, 1987

21. Gunne LM, Growdon J, Glaeser B: Oral dyskinesia in rats following brain lesions and neuroleptic drug administration. Psychopharmacology 77:134–139, 1982

22. Mithani S, Atmadja S, Baimbridge KG, et al: Neuroleptic-induced oral dyskinesias: effects of progabide and lack of correlation with regional changes in glutamic acid decarboxylase and choline acetyltransferase activities. Psychopharmacology 93:94–100, 1987

23. Casey DE, Gerlach J, Magelund G, et al: Gamma-acetylenic GABA in tardive dyskinesia. Arch Gen Psychiatry 37:1376–1379, 1980

24. Korsgaard S, Casey DE, Gerlach J: Effect of gamma-vinyl GABA in tardive dyskinesia. Psychiatry Res 8:261–269, 1983

25. Stahl SM, Thornton JE, Simpson ML, et al. Gamma-vinyl GABA treatment of tardive dyskinesia and other movement disorders. Biol. Psychiatry 20:888–893, 1985

26. Tamminga CA, Thaker GT, Hare T, et al: GABA agonist therapy improves tardive dyskinesia. Lancet 2:97–98, 1983

27. Tell GP, Schechter PJ, Koch-Weser J, et al: Effects of gamma-vinyl GABA. N Engl J Med 305:581–582, 1981

28. Alphs LD, Davis JM: Treatments for tardive dyskinesia: an overview of noncatecholaminergic/noncholinergic treatments, in Movement Disorders. Edited by Shaw NS, Donald AG. New York, Plenum, 1986, pp. 205–226

29. Tamminga CA, Crayton JW, Chase TN: Improvement in tardive dyskinesia after muscimol therapy. Arch Gen Psychiatry 36:595–598, 1979

30. Morselli PL, Bossi L, Henry JF, et al: On the therapeutic action of SL 76002, a new GABA-neurotransmission drug. Brain Res Bull 5 (Suppl 2):411–414, 1980

31. Singh MM, Becker RE, Pitman RK, et al: Diazepam-induced changes in tardive dyskinesia: suggestions for a new conceptual model. Biol Psychiatry 17:729–742, 1982

32. Chien C, Jung K, Ross-Townsent A: Efficacies of agents related to GABA, dopamine and acetylcholine in the treatment of tardive dyskinesia. Psychopharmacol Bull 14:20–22, 1978

33. Gerlach J, Rye T, Kristjansen P: Effect of baclofen on tardive dyskinesia. Psychopharmacology 56:145–151, 1978

34. Glazer WM, Moore DC, Bowers MB, et al: The treatment of tardive dyskinesia with baclofen. Psychopharmacology 87:480–483, 1985

35. Nair VNP, Yassa R, Ruiz-Navarro J, et al: Baclofen in the treatment of tardive dyskinesia. Am J Psychiatry 135:1562–1563, 1978

36. Simpson GM, Lee HJ, Shrivastava RK, et al: Baclofen in the treatment of tardive dyskinesia and schizophrenia. Psychopharmacol Bull 14:16–18, 1978

37. Gibson A: Sodium valproate and tardive dyskinesia. Br J Psychiatry 133:82, 1978

38. Linnoila M, Viukari M, Hietala O: Effect of sodium valproate on tardive dyskinesia. Br J Psychiatry 129:114–119, 1976

39. Lloyd KG, Hornykiewicz O: Effect of chronic neuroleptic or L-dopa administration on GABA levels in the rat substantia nigra. Life Sci 21:1489–1496, 1977

40. Rupniak NMJ, Prestwich SA, Horton RW, et al: Alterations in cerebral glutamic acid decarboxylase and ^{3}H-flunitrazepam binding during continuous treatment of rats for up to 1 year with haloperidol, sulpiride or clozapine. J Neural Transm 68:113–125, 1987

Chapter 4

Neuroendocrine and Cerebrospinal Measurements in Schizophrenic Patients with Tardive Dyskinesia

Michael Davidson, M.D.
Miklos F. Losonczy, M.D., Ph.D.
Richard C. Mohs, Ph.D.
Bonnie M. Davis, M.D.
Theresa A. Ryan, B.S.
Richard S. E. Keefe
Kenneth L. Davis, M.D.

Chapter 4

*Neuroendocrine and
Cerebrospinal Measurements
in Schizophrenic Patients
with Tardive Dyskinesia*

Clinical observations suggest that tardive dyskinesia (TD) is associated with a state of dopamine (DA) hyperactivity. Dopaminergic agents such as L-dopa and amphetamine aggravate symptoms of TD (1, 2), while DA-depleting agents and DA receptor blockers decrease the frequency of dyskinetic movements (3). A DA receptor supersensitivity hypothesis has been invoked to explain the paradoxical situation in which neuroleptic drugs, known to inhibit dopaminergic activity acutely, ultimately increase dopaminergic activity and predispose to TD. According to this hypothesis, chronic receptor blockade or "chemical denervation" induces receptor proliferation and consequently augments the responsiveness to DA, manifested as dopaminergic hyperactivity. Indeed chronic administration of neuroleptics to rodents does increase the number of dopaminergic binding sites and augments movements thought to reflect dopaminergic neurotransmission following a challenge with a DA agonist (4). Similarly, increased numbers of dopaminergic binding sites have been reported in brain tissue from schizophrenic patients chronically treated with neuroleptics. The evidence supporting a role for a hyperdopaminergic state in patients with TD is presently circumstantial. Clinical attempts to demonstrate DA receptor supersensitivity have focused on measuring plasma levels of anterior pituitary hormones and cerebrospinal concentrations of DA metabolites and cyclic nucleotides linked to DA neurotransmission.

Dopaminergic mechanisms modulate growth hormone (GH) and prolactin (PRL) release, increasing GH secretion and suppressing PRL. If pituitary DA receptors become supersensitive in schizo-

41

phrenic patients with TD, then these patients could have an increased tonic secretion of GH and enhanced suppression of PRL compared to patients without TD. However, studies in which PRL or GH plasma levels were compared between schizophrenic patients with and without TD have failed to distinguish between the two groups (5–11). As a test to the supersensitivity hypothesis, these findings are inconclusive since plasma GH and PRL levels reflect tuberoinfundibular dopaminergic activity and not the nigrostriatal dopaminergic activity that is presumably more relevant for movement disorders.

A more pertinent measure may be the cerebrospinal fluid (CSF) homovanillic acid (HVA) concentration, which predominantly reflects the dopaminergic activity of nigrostriatal neurons. Dopamine receptor supersensitivity in the caudate would be expected to induce a decrease in DA turnover reflected by reduced CSF HVA concentrations. Reduced CSF HVA concentrations in patients with TD was suggested by one study (12) but not found in four others (13–15). These conflicting results are not surprising. Measurements of CSF HVA and/or GH and PRL plasma levels have serious methodological problems that limit their utility as indicators of DA activity. GH and PRL concentrations can be affected by age, weight, and factors related to the experimental environment like length of hospitalization, stress, physical activity, and diet. Similarly, CSF HVA concentrations are affected by age, height, physical activity, and seasonal rhythms. Moreover, both neuroendocrine and CSF studies in TD patients have often been flawed by the selection of inappropriate control subjects.

The current study was an attempt to elaborate possible in vivo evidence of DA receptor supersensitivity in TD through CSF and neuroendocrine approaches with particular emphasis to the control of confounding factors that could affect these measurements. GH, PRL, and CSF HVA values were compared between schizophrenic patients with and without TD.

METHOD

Subjects were 31 schizophrenic inpatients, 14 of whom scored 2 or more points on two of the first four items of the Abnormal Involuntary Movement Scale (AIMS) and 17 of whom were without abnormal movements. The mean ± SEM age for the TD group was 45 ± 4 and 34.9 ± 3 for the non-TD group. Diagnoses of schizophrenia were made by consensus by two experienced clinicians using the Schedule for Affective Disorders, and meeting either Research Diagnostic Criteria or Feighner criteria for chronic schizophrenia.

Severity of the schizophrenic illness reflected by Brief Psychiatric Rating Scale scores was similar for the TD and non-TD group (means = 38 and 34, respectively). The diagnosis of TD was based on the AIMS scores assigned by two independent raters observing the same rating session. The interrater reliability coefficient for AIMS was .85. All patients were rated at least three times during a 1-week period in the same position and room under similar environmental conditions (light and noise). At the time of the rating patients had been drug free for at least 2 weeks (TD mean = 23 days, SD = ± 4; non-TD mean = 21 days, SD = ± 5) and received no depot neuroleptics for the last 3 months. The possibility that PRL, GH, and CSF HVA differences might be apparent only between clearly distinct groups would suggest that criteria for TD or absence of abnormal movements should be more restrictive than generally accepted in the research literature (16). TD was diagnosed in patients whom both raters assigned at least a score of 2 on two of the first four AIMS items. The non-TD group included patients in whom AIMS scores assigned by both raters on the same first four times did not exceed 1. Patients were hospitalized 2 weeks prior to the study and consumed a standard low-monoamine diet for the same period. Probenecid 100 mg/kg was administered to all subjects in divided doses at 20.00h, 01.00h, 05.00h, 08.00h, 11.00h and the lumbar puncture was performed in a recumbent position at 14.00h following approximately 15 hours of bed rest. An intravenous catheter was inserted at 08.00h and blood samples for GH and PRL were drawn every 20 minutes between 08.45 and 12.45h. HVA and probenecid concentrations were measured from standardized CSF aliquots, which were frozen upon withdrawal. HVA and probenecid were assayed by high pressure liquid chromatography (HPLC), and PRL and GH were assayed by radioimmunoassay (RIA). Statistical calculations were performed with SPSS Software, using an analysis of covariance covarying for age, weight, and probenecid concentration where applicable.

RESULTS AND DISCUSSION

As evident from Table 1 mean plasma concentrations of PRL throughout the 4-hour procedure were significantly lower in patients with a diagnosis of chronic schizophrenia and TD than in patients without TD. Plasma GH concentrations or CSF HVA concentrations did not distinguish between schizophrenic patients with or without TD (see Table 2).

Although the finding that concentrations of PRL were lower in the TD group may be consistent with the hypothesis that TD is a

Table 1. PRL and GH values in TD and non-TD patients*

	PRL	GH
TD schizophrenics	2.8 ng/ml ±.50 (n=14)	3.0 ng/ml±.69 (n=10)
Non-TD schizophrenics	5.4 ng/ml ±.94 (n=17)	5.5 ng/ml ±.81 (n=13)

*Values covaried for age and weight
1) Mean average PRL TD versus non-TD F (5.90) = 1,27,p <.02
2) Mean average GH saline, TD versus non-TD F (.04) = 1, 20, p = .83

Table 2. CSF HVA and cAMP values in TD and non-TD patients*

	CSF HVA
TD schizophrenics	240.4 ng/ml ±43 (n=8)
Non-TD schizophrenics	227.1 ng/ml ±24 (n=12)

*Values covaried for probenecid concentrations
Mean CSF HVA concentrations TD versus non-TD F (.17) = 1, 15, p = .68

manifestation of DA receptor supersensitivity, that is not the only possible explanation. It might superficially appear somewhat surprising that differences were found in PRL concentrations, but not GH concentrations. However, numerous differences exist in the control of these systems. For example, DA receptors for the lactotropic cells lie totally outside the blood–brain barrier, whereas dopaminergic effects on GH concentrations are mediated by events both within and outside the blood–brain barrier. Conceivably, higher concentrations of neuroleptic outside than inside the brain could expose the dopaminergic receptor mediating PRL release to higher concentrations of neuroleptic than might occur to dopaminergic receptors linked to GH. Furthermore, a number of neurotransmitter systems affect one of these hormones without affecting the other, and it might be naive to conceive of the chronic effects of neuroleptics on neurotransmission as solely related to DA. As TD is thought to be more closely related to the nigrostriatal dopaminergic tract than the tuberoinfundibular, the more obvious site to have reflected a hyperdopaminergic state in TD was the nigrostriatal system, and this should have been reflected in CSF HVA. However, there was no difference, not even a trend, for HVA concentrations between the TD and non-TD group.

Postmortem studies indicate that chronic schizophrenic patients, compared to normal controls, have increased numbers of dopamine binding sites in several brain regions. Whether this difference is a function of chronic exposure to neuroleptics or a manifestation of schizophrenia itself remains unresolved. However, it does seem certain that the proliferation of DA receptors seen on autopsy is far more prevalent than is the prevalence of TD in that population. It is conceivable that DA receptor supersensitivity, as reflected in increased binding, is common to the vast majority of schizophrenic patients who have received chronic neuroleptic therapy, but that only those schizophrenic patients who lack other compensatory mechanisms in other neurotransmitter systems manifest abnormal involuntary movements. In that case, CSF HVA levels might be lower in all schizophrenic patients treated with chronic neuroleptics than in normal controls. Indeed, when all the schizophrenic patients in the current study were compared to normal controls, their CSF HVA levels were, as a group, significantly lower than those of a matched control population (K.L. Davis, unpublished data, 1987).

Yet another factor may have mitigated against finding differences in CSF HVA. Probenecid is used to block the outflow of HVA from the CSF in order to amplify dopaminergic turnover. This technique makes the assumption that at high levels of probenecid concentration there is almost complete blockage of HVA efflux. It is, however, recognized that this is not the case and that the effects of probenecid, depending on the concentrations of probenecid achieved in the CSF of each patient, can be variable.

Hence, for reasons that remain somewhat unclear, PRL concentrations may be more sensitive to neuroleptic-induced alterations of dopaminergic neurotransmission than other markers of dopaminergic activity. It might therefore be of substantial interest to follow concentrations of PRL in patients at risk for TD in order to determine the temporal relationship of PRL lowering to the earliest manifestation of this disorder.

REFERENCES

1. Hippius H, Longemann G: Zur wirkung von dioxyphenylalanin (L-dope) auf extrapyramidal motorische hyperkinesen nach langfristiger neuroleptischer therapie. Arzneimittel-Forschung 20:894–896, 1970

2. Carroll BJ, Curtis GC, Keekmen E: Paradoxical response to dopamine agonists in tardive dyskinesia. Am J Psychiatry 1134:785–789, 1977

3. Kazmatsuri H, Chien C, Cole JO: Therapeutic approaches to tardive dyskinesia. Arch Gen Psychiatry 27:491–499, 1972

4. Rastogi SK, Rastogi RB, Singhai RL, et al: Behavioral and biochemical alteration following haloperidol treatment and withdrawal: the animal model of tardive dyskinesia reexamined. Prog Neuropsychopharmacol Biol Psychiatry 7:153–164, 1983

5. Ettigi P, Nair NPV, Cerbantes P: Effect of apomorphine on growth hormone and prolactin secretion in schizophrenic patients with and without oral dyskinesia withdrawn from chronic neuroleptic therapy. Arch Gen Psychiatry 321:870–876, 1976

6. Meltzer HY, Goode DJ, Fang VS et al: Dopamine and schizophrenia. Lancet 2:1142, 1976

7. Tamminga CA, Smith RE, Pandey G, et al: A neuroendocrine study of supersensitivity in tardive dyskinesia. Arch Gen Psychiatry 34:1199–1203, 1977

8. Asnis GM, Sachar EJ, Langer G, et al: Normal prolactin response in tardive dyskinesia. Psychopharmacology 66:247–250, 1979

9. Cohen KL, Cooper RA, Alsthul S: Prolactin levels in tardive dyskinesia. N Engl J Med 300:46, 1979

10. Jeste DV, Neckers LM, Wagner RL, et al: Lymphocytes monoamine oxidase and plasma prolactin and growth hormone in tardive dyskinesia. J Clin Psychiatry 42:75–77, 1981

11. Chase TN, Shur JA, Gordon EK: Cerebrospinal fluid monoamine metabolites in drug induced extrapyramidal disorders. Neuropharmacology 9:265–268, 1970

12. Pind K, Faurbye A: Concentration of homovanillic acid in cerebrospinal fluid after treatment with probenecid in patients with drug induced tardive dyskinesia. Acta Psychiatr Scand 46:323–326, 1970

13. Curzon G: Involuntary movements other than parkinsonism: biochemical aspects. Proc R Soc Med 66:873–876, 1973

14. Bowers MD, Jr., Moore D, Tarsy D: Tardive dyskinesia: a clinical test of supersensitivity hypothesis. Psychopharmacology 61:137–141, 1979

15. Nagao T, Oshino T, Misunolobu K, et al: Cerebrospinal fluid monoamine metabolites and cyclic nucleotides in chronic schizophrenic patients with tardive dyskinesia or drug induced tremor. Biol Psychiatry 14:509–523, 1979

16. Schooler NR, Kane JM: Research diagnosis criteria for tardive dyskinesia. Arch Gen Psychiatry 39:486–487, 1982

Chapter 5

Abnormal Involuntary Movements and Psychosis in the Preneuroleptic Era and in Unmedicated Patients: Implications for the Concept of Tardive Dyskinesia

John L. Waddington, M.A., Ph.D.
Timothy J. Crow, Ph.D., F.R.C. Psych.

Chapter 5

Abnormal Involuntary Movements and Psychosis in the Preneuroleptic Era and in Unmedicated Patients: Implications for the Concept of Tardive Dyskinesia

The phenomenology, epidemiology, pharmacology, and putative pathophysiology of tardive dyskinesia have been well documented (1–5). This syndrome of abnormal, involuntary choreoathetoid movements affects principally the orobuccolingual and facial area but sometimes extends to limbs and trunk. It is widely regarded as a debilitating consequence of neuroleptic drug exposure, occurring in 20 to 25 percent of patients after several years of treatment. Though this syndrome has been documented in several diagnostic groups, it has been most extensively studied in schizophrenia. Because of the ubiquitous use of neuroleptic drugs for more than a quarter century, a vital issue for the above concept is the extent to which such abnormal, involuntary movements were seen in schizophrenic patients before the advent of neuroleptics. In the modern era, a few authors (6, 7) have drawn attention to earlier historical reports of apparently similar movements in schizophrenic patients. However, recent reviewers have failed to locate qualitative descriptions and quantitative prevalence estimates of such movements in the preneuroleptic era. This, together with a progressive increase in the reported prevalence of abnormal, involuntary movements in neuroleptic-treated populations since the introduction of neuroleptic drugs, has been offered as firm evidence that tardive dyskinesia is neuroleptic dependent (1, 2).

A recent survey of the movement status of a population of chronic schizophrenic patients never treated with neuroleptics (8) prompted us to reevaluate the literature on this topic. We have located many qualitative and some quantitative reports of abnormal, involuntary choreoathetoid movements in schizophrenic patients in the preneuroleptic era.

QUALITATIVE REPORTS

The presence of choreiform movements in psychiatric patients has been recognized since at least 1845. A review (9) of this very early literature written before the identification of schizophrenia (dementia praecox) as a nosological entity recognized that insanity and chorea could coexist in a single individual. Diller (9) noted the importance of distinguishing such individuals from those suffering from rheumatic (that is, Sydenham's) or heredity (that is, Huntington's) chorea. He wrote that "In all long-standing cases of chorea there is a more or less marked tendency to mental deterioration which, in many cases, progressively increases and finally terminates in dementia." And that "A person having a family history of insanity, chorea or epilepsy or indeed any nervous affliction, is predisposed to an attack of chorea." However, whether Diller used the term *chorea* with the wider connotation that it has today and whether insanity as he described it included patients who would now be described as suffering from psychosis is unclear.

The first systematic description of abnormal movements in schizophrenia is that of Kraepelin (10). He described "the spasmodic phenomena in the musculature of the face . . . , distortion of the corners of the mouth, irregular movements of the tongue and lips. . . . They remind one of the corresponding disorder of choreic patients. . . . Connected with these are further smacking and clicking of the tongue. . . . Several patients continually carried out peculiar sprawling, irregular choreiform outspreading movements which I think I can best characterize by the expression 'athetoid ataxia.'"

Similarly, Bleuler (11) described "tremulous and wavering" in schizophrenia. He refers to "extraordinary movements of tongue and lips. . . . All these peculiarities are the reasons why some authors have spoken of choreic or tetanic movements in catatonia" (pp. 94–226). Bleuler felt that such movements could be better explained as psychological than as neurological phenomena. For example he described pursing and pouting of the lips, a common component of the "tardive dyskinesia" syndrome, but felt these were more readily understood as an expression of contempt than as an involuntary contradiction of the muscles controlling protrusion of the lips. At another point Bleuler (11) wrote "Fibrillary contractions are particularly noticeable in the facial muscles" (p. 170), and "'sheet lighting' (as this phenomenon is called) has long been known as a sign of chronically developing illness. Contractions of single muscles or of entire limbs are observed more rarely" (p. 170).

Choreiform movements in schizophrenia were further described by Farran-Ridge (12), who noted that patients "purse the lips, distort the angles of the mouth, and make irregular movements of the tongue in such a way as to remind one strongly, as Kraepelin long ago pointed out, of the corresponding disorders of choreic patients." Similarly, Reiter (13) presented case studies in schizophrenia and in individual patients noting "choreatic, athetotic movements," "choreatic, athetotic restlessness of both hands," and that "the spasms continue and have, especially as far as his face is concerned, increased; round the mouth they are now of the chorea Huntington type . . . more particularly, in the muscles of mastication with incessant smacking of the lips . . . and some choreatic restlessness in his arms." More detailed descriptions of abnormal, involuntary movements in schizophrenia by Jelliffe (14) include "Blowing out of the cheeks, rubbing the nose or face, tongue plays and the thousand and one minor and major apparently senseless movement of face, neck, shoulders, arm, fingers, trunk, legs, toes, etc."

Measurement of spontaneous movements in 150 adult psychotic patients by Jones (15), using a time-sample technique, detected oral movements that "included lip pursing, lip sucking, finger or thumb sucking, protrusion of the tongue and lip licking." Unfortunately, as with the other studies noted above, no quantitative measures were made and no prevalence estimates are available. These studies can serve only as striking qualitative descriptions to set alongside views on the clinical features of tardive dyskinesia.

QUANTITATIVE STUDIES

If the above descriptions of abnormal, involuntary, choreoathetoid movements in schizophrenia are genuinely representative of an as yet unspecified proportion of patients, one might expect them to be apparent in the classifications of schizophrenia proposed by psychiatrists wishing to obtain clear concepts of individual abnormal phenomena. The classification of schizophrenia proposed by Leonhard (16, 17) was derived from that of his colleague Kleist and was introduced from the German into the English-language literature by Fish (18). Within this system, the abnormal, involuntary choreoathetoid movements in schizophrenia described above are regarded as being of sufficient prevalence and prominence to define the subtype of "parakinetic catatonia." Fish (18), translated the characteristics of this form of schizophrenia as follows: "Thus parakinetic catatonia resembles chorea. . . . Voluntary actions are carried out in an unnatural awkward way and involuntary movements are jerky and reminiscent of choreiform movements. . . . The involuntary movements which occur seem to be distorted reactive and pseudo-expressive movements. Facial movements are especially affected." Leonhard's parakinetic catatonic therefore appears to be no more than an attempt to define a type of schizophrenia by the presence of the simple involuntary choreathetoid movements as described by Kraepelin, Bleuler, and others.

Leonhard (16) examined 400 patients with chronic "systemic" (that is, unequivocal and symptomatologically consistent) schizophrenia. Of these, 35 were classified as parakinetic catatonic (7.9 percent). Later, Leonhard (17) examined a further 324 patients with systemic schizophrenia, of whom he classified 17 (5.2 percent) as having parakinetic catatonia. In addition to introducing this classification to the English literature, Fish (18) himself applied it to a population of English patients. In his investigation of 95 patients with chronic systemic schizophrenia, he found 5 (5.3 percent) to have parakinetic catatonia. This study was begun in 1955, before the widespread introduction of neuroleptics. In 1964, Fish (19) reported on a Swedish population of 351 chronic systemic schizophrenic patients who had been studied, in association with Astrup, before and after commencing treatment with neuroleptics. Of these, 18 (5.1 percent) showed parakinetic catatonia before neuroleptic treatment (Table 1).

The study of Yarden and DiScipio (6) is also relevant. These authors investigated consecutive first-admission schizophrenic pa-

Table 1. Prevalence of choreoathetoid movements in schizophrenic populations not exposed to neuroleptics.

Study	Year	Total n	Dyskinesia n	%
Leonhard	1936	400	35	7.9
Leonhard	1957	324	17	5.2
Fish	1958	95	5	5.3
Fish	1964	351	18	5.1
Yarden and DiScipio	1971	275	18	6.5

tients for choreiform and athetoid movements and identified 18 such patients (mean age, 24 years). Though they did not report the number of schizophrenic patients screened to isolate this group with abnormal, involuntary choreathetoid movements, a personal communication from these authors clarified that between 250 and 300 patients were seen over a 1-year period. Therefore, the prevalence of abnormal, involuntary movements in their sample was approximately 6.5 percent. This figure is contrasted in Table 1 with those from the above studies of parakinetic catatonia.

RELATIONSHIP TO TARDIVE DYSKINESIA

The presence of abnormal, involuntary choreoathetoid movements in schizophrenic patients in the preneuroleptic era prompts the question as to whether or not these movements share characteristics with those that today are described as "tardive dyskinesia." This question may be answered by the following comparisons:

Phenomenology

It has been suggested by some (20) that these early descriptions of abnormal movements represent the classical stereotypies and mannerisms of schizophrenia rather than true choreoathetoid dyskinesia. However, both Kraepelin (10) and Bleuler (11) gave careful descriptions of motor and other phenomena in schizophrenia and distinguished between choreiform movements and stereotypies or mannerisms. It is important also to note that Kleist's and Leonhard's classifications of schizophrenia specifically dissociated parakinetic (choreiform) catatonia from manneristic catatonia, in which stereotypies are seen (16, 17).

Yarden and DiScipio (6) again clearly distinguished between abnormal, choreoathetoid movements and the usual stereotypies and mannerisms of schizophrenia. If the above descriptions are compared with those of the comprehensive Rockland Scale of Simpson et al. (21) for tardive dyskinesia, it is difficult to avoid the conclusion that such patients satisfy criteria for this diagnosis. Some modern investigators have acknowledged this. Thus Jeste and Wyatt (2) agree that dyskinesia existed in the preneuroleptic era and concede that the important question is whether a tardive dyskinesia-like syndrome was as prevalent then as it is today.

Neuroleptic Sensitivity

The abnormal, involuntary movements of tardive dyskinesia are often suppressed, at least temporarily, by increasing the dose of the neuroleptic that is presumed to have caused the dyskinesia or by reintroducing neuroleptics if previously withdrawn (3). The abnormal, involuntary movements described in the preneuroleptic era show a similar sensitivity to attenuation by neuroleptics. Fish (19) reported that the parakinesia of parakinetic (choreiform) catatonia was improved after initiating neuroleptic treatment. However, none of the patients was rated as showing the considerable improvement with neuroleptics noted in other groups; this is in agreement with the report of Yarden and DiScipio (6). Therefore the abnormal movements of the preneuroleptic era share with tardive dyskinesia a degree of neuroleptic sensitivity.

Exacerbation by Stress

It is commonly accepted that intensity of tardive dyskinesia is not constant but modulated by psychosocial influences, for example, stress (20). Bleuler (11) reported abnormal movements in schizophrenia to change in intensity under psychic influence from zero to maximum. Similarly, Fish (18) and Leonhard (17) noted that parakinetic (choreiform) hyperkinesias became more pronounced when the patient was "stimulated."

Prognostic Significance

Kucharski et al. (22) evaluated the discharge status of 265 inpatients with tardive dyskinesia over a 2-year period. Those not discharged had significantly higher ratings of abnormal movements and earlier age at first hospitalization than those discharged. Moreover Chouinard et al. (23) found length of hospitalization and resistance to treatment to be associated with tardive dyskinesia. It is striking that Kraepelin (10), Bleuler (11), and Fish (18, 19) reported abnormal movements in schizophrenia to be associated with a poor prognosis and response to treatment. Similarly, Yarden and DiScipio (6) reported choreoathetoid movements in young first admissions to their unit to be associated with earlier age at first hospitalization, poor response to treatment, and nondischarge.

Age

It is commonly stated that abnormal, involuntary movements, especially those of the orofacial region, emerge in non-neuroleptic-treated patients as a consequence of aging processes (2, 4, 24). However, most studies on elderly nonschizophrenic populations are confounded by overt or occult neuropsychiatric disorder and/or poor documentation of absence of neuroleptic treatment. To our knowledge, only two modern studies have systematically evaluated the prevalence of abnormal, involuntary movements in large populations of normal elderly subjects specifically selected for the absence both of any neuropsychiatric history and of neuroleptic exposure. Klawans and Barr (25) reported that 2 of 238 subjects (0.8 percent) ages 50 to 59 years and 29 of 423 subjects (6.8 percent) ages 60 to 79 showed orofacial dyskinesia. Similarly Kane et al. (26) reported that 5 of 127 subjects (4 percent) (mean age, 72 years) showed abnormal movements, predominantly of the orofacial region.

If reports of such movements in the preneuroleptic era were derived principally from studies of elderly schizophrenic patients, they may simply reflect this spontaneous dyskinesia of aging. However, in Fish's study (19) geriatric patients were specifically excluded. Also the schizophrenic patients of Reiter (13) with choreoathetoid movements were ages 36 to 61 years, and Yarden and DiScipio (6) studied patients with a mean age of 24 years. Thus it is clear we are not dealing with an effect attributable to normal aging processes.

RELATIONSHIP TO MODERN STUDIES AND SPECIFICITY FOR SCHIZOPHRENIA

These five early studies (Table 1) indicate that a syndrome of abnormal, involuntary choreoathetoid movements occurred at least in schizophrenia before the introduction of neuroleptics. Despite their diversity (with regard to era, country of origin, criteria, and patient population) they are remarkably consistent in their estimates of the prevalence of such abnormal movements (mean ± SD, 6.0% ± 0.5 of 1,485 schizophrenic patients). A recent review (4) of dyskinesia in 56 diverse neuroleptic-treated populations indicates a considerably higher prevalence (mean ± SD, 20.0% ± 1.9 of 34,552 patients). While the five early studies (6, 16–19) were performed between 1936 and 1971, these later neuroleptic studies were carried out between 1960 and 1980, and include organic and other diagnoses in addition to schizophrenia. Because recent heightened awareness of dyskinesia and the introduction of systematic rating scales might lower the threshold for its detection, and because of patient heterogeneity, it may not be valid to compare these differing prevalence estimates of dyskinesia. This point can be clarified in recent studies using such systematic rating scales on populations of schizophrenic patients who had and had not received neuroleptics.

Brandon et al. (27) examined the 910 inmates of a regional mental hospital who had been resident for a period of more than 3 months for the bucco-linguo-masticatory triad and did not find impressively significant differences in incidence between phenothiazine-treated and nontreated patients in several age and sex groups. However, the patient population in this study is heterogeneous with respect to diagnosis and no quantitative assessment of abnormal movements was made. More directly relevant is the study of Owens et al. (8), who examined the prevalence of movement disorder with the Abnormal Involuntary Movement Scale (AIMS) in the population of patients with a diagnosis of schizophrenia according to St. Louis criteria in an area mental hospital in Northwest London. Included in this population was a group of 47 patients who on account of the treatment practices of the medical staff (who, under the influence of R. D. Laing, for a number of years favored a therapeutic community approach to the treatment of psychosis) had never received neuroleptic medication. The prevalence of abnormal movements was similar in patients who had not received medication and in those who were currently receiving or had previously received such drugs, although when age was taken into account the prevalence of abnormal movements was found increased in those who had received medication. No differences in the distribution of form of abnormal movements were detected between the groups of patients who had and had not received neuroleptic medication.

More recently, Waddington et al. (28) examined a small number of similarly diagnosed chronic schizophrenic patients who had remained free from neuroleptic treatment. The reasons why these elderly patients, all in their ninth decade of life, had not been exposed to neuroleptics differed from those applying to the sample of Owens and colleagues (8). The clinical picture in this subgroup was characteristic of the "defect state" of schizophrenia, florid positive symptoms having abated before the introduction of neuroleptics, and the potential dangers of neuroleptic treatment having been judged to outweigh the small likelihood of any therapeutic improvement being derived. These patients were matched with a similar schizophrenic group (of comparable age) but with a history of long-term neuroleptic treatment and were further subdivided on the basis of whether or not they were currently receiving neuroleptics. Abnormal movements were observed in all three groups; there were no significant differences in scores on the AIMS between patients who had and had not been exposed to neuroleptics, and this lack of difference could not be accounted for in terms of current neuroleptic treatment. We have not been able to locate any similar studies on the baseline level of movement disorder in patients with affective disorder.

IS PERSISTENT DYSKINESIA DUE TO NEUROLEPTIC DRUGS?

These findings establish clearly, as is apparent from the historical record of the preneuroleptic era, that abnormal involuntary movement indistinguishable from those now described as tardive dyskinesia occur in patients with schizophrenia who have not received neuroleptic medication. This conclusion casts considerable doubt on prevailing practice that attributes all abnormal involuntary movements in patients with schizophrenia to the effects of long-term neuroleptic medication (29). This clearly cannot be the case. The question rather is what proportion of such abnormal involuntary movements might be so attributable and, more importantly from a clinical and legal perspective, whether an irreversible component of such movements can be attributed to neuroleptic medication.

It seems clear that drugs do sometimes induce movements—it is a common clinical observation that some patients lose much movements in the period following drug discontinuation. Although neither phenomenon is authenticated by controlled observations of the type that have established the therapeutic efficacy of neuroleptic drugs, such changes, together with the sensitivity of some established dyskinesias to attenuation by acute neuroleptic challenge, have contributed greatly to the plausibility of the view that dyskinesias are caused by neuroleptic drugs. The central question, however, remains whether neuroleptic drugs induce irreversible movement changes.

The literature we have reviewed emphasizes how exceedingly difficult it is in either an individual or the general case to determine whether persisting abnormal movements are truly drug induced. The fact that such movements persist after drug withdrawal constitutes no evidence for such a presumption because it is entirely possible that in a particular case persisting movements are disease related and would have been present even if neuroleptic drugs had never been given.

Studies on the prevalence of abnormal movements in patients on and off medication are unlikely to clarify this issue. First, the clinician's decision on whether to medicate is unlikely to be independent of the risk of abnormal movements; for example, patients with severe schizophrenic illnesses who might also be at greater risk of disease-related dyskinesias may be more likely to be treated with high doses of neuroleptic drugs, and conversely, at least in recent years, these drugs are more likely to be reduced or withdrawn if abnormal movements are seen. Moreover the drugs while they are administered may affect the movements themselves, either suppressing them or occasionally exacerbating them. These factors militate against unequivocal information concerning the role of drugs being obtained from comparisons between patient groups whose drug administration has not been treated as an experimental variable. Only a long-term trial in which patients were allocated to neuroleptics or placebo from an early stage of illness and the drug-treated group were subsequently withdrawn could answer this question. A significant excess of dyskinetic movements persisting after drug withdrawal in the drug-treated group would establish the tardive dyskinesia hypothesis. However, in such a trial it would be required that the sample size exceeds that of studies of the therapeutic effect by the ratio of "drug responsive" to the postulated dyskinesia-susceptible patients, and the duration exceeds that of the period over which it is predicted the drug-induced dyskinesia develops. Such a trial presents substantial practical and ethical problems.

CLINICAL CORRELATES OF DYSKINESIA

The literature we have reviewed casts considerable doubt on the view that all abnormal involuntary movements in schizophrenia, commonly referred to as tardive dyskinesia, are due to neuroleptic drug administration. Clearly movements identical in form to those described as tardive dyskinesia occur in patients who have not received such drugs. When present they may be modulated by neuroleptic drugs, but the case that an irreversible component of such dyskinesias is attributable to drugs has yet to be established.

The alternative view is that the persistent component of such movements is associated with a disease process, and especially, that it is preferentially related to types of psychotic illness associated with poor prognosis. Thus the parakinetic catatonia of Kleist is included by him among the "systemic" types of schizophrenia, which he regards as of more insidious onset and steadily progressive course than the "non-systemic" schizophrenias (for example, "affect-laden paraphrenia," "schizophasia," and periodic catatonia"). A simpler typology that has attracted recent attention is based on the distinction between positive and negative symptoms. Positive symptoms are delusions, hallucinations, and thought disorder, features that are pathological by their presence. Negative symptoms include flattening of affect and poverty of speech, features that are pathological because some normal function is lost. It is suggested (30) that these groups of symptoms can be used to define two syndromes and that these reflect different aspects of the disease process. Positive symptoms occur typically in acute episodes and negative symptoms in chronic states—but of course both types of symptoms occur in either situation and they can certainly occur together. Positive symptoms predict potential response to neuroleptic medication; negative symptoms respond much less well and appear more closely associated with poor long-term outcome—they are sometimes, perhaps often, associated with the intellectual impairment that increasingly is recognized as a component of the defect syndrome. It is postulated that the two syndromes related to different aspects of the underlying disease process—the first syndrome to a neurochemical disturbance (perhaps an increase in numbers of dopamine-2 receptors, which would account for the response of positive symptoms to dopamine antagonist drugs), the second syndrome to cell loss and the consequent structural changes that have been identified by pneumoencephalography, x-ray computed tomography, and postmortem studies. Thus the two syndromes may reflect reversible and irreversible components of the disease process (30, 31).

Over the past few years, an increasing number of studies have indicated that schizophrenic patients with involuntary movements are characterized by greater cognitive dysfunction, negative symptoms, and abnormalities in brain morphology than otherwise indistinguishable patients without such movements, and there is one report of a similar association with cognitive dysfunction in bipolar patients (for a review see Waddington (32)). These findings are consistent with the view that dyskinesias, at least those occurring in schizophrenia, are related to those features of the illness that are associated with poor outcome and structural brain pathology.

CONCLUSION

A crucial question is whether these phenomena are specific for schizophrenia and other psychotic disorders or reflect the structural brain changes that occur in classical organic (for example, dementing) illnesses. The literature on the prevalence of abnormal movements in various patient groups not exposed to neuroleptics is usually considered to be highly inconsistent (range = 0 to 39 percent; see Kane and Smith (4)). However, the findings are more uniform when one subdivides such studies by inclusion or exclusion of dementia from the study population. Thus Martinelli and Gabellini (33) found abnormal orofacial movements in 7.7 percent of 104 patients up to 84 years old who showed essential tremor, indistinguishable from the prevalence in the normal elderly population (26, 25) (Table 2). Conversely, four studies (27, 34–36) in which an (unspecified) proportion of cases showed clinical evidence of dementia, among other mixed neurological signs, have reported high prevalences of abnormal orofacial movements (18 to 38 percent) in substantial populations of older patients for whom a history of exposure to neuroleptics had been excluded. Molsa et al. (37, 38) have recently reported involuntary orofacial movements in 16.8 percent of 143 patients with Alzheimer's disease who were not exposed to neuroleptics.

It should be emphasized that when abnormal movements have

Table 2. Prevalence of orofacial dyskinesia in elderly populations not exposed to neuroleptics, with and without central nervous system (CNS) disorder.

Study	Year	CNS disorder	Age	Total n	Dyskinesia n	%
Neuroleptic exposure and CNS disorder excluded						
Klawans and Barr	1982	—	50–59	238	2	0.8
			60–69	233	14	6.0
			70–79	190	15	7.8
Kane et al.	1982	—	73±7	127	5	4.0
Neuroleptic exposure excluded						
Martinelli and Gabellini	1982	Essential tremor	65–84	104	8	7.7
Molsa et al.	1982	Arteriosclerotic dementia	45–85 +	91	11	12.1
Molsa et al.	1984	Alzheimer dementia	45–85 +	143	24	16.8
Bourgeois et al.	1980	Mixed, incl. dementia	76	211	36	17.1
Blowers	1981	Mixed, incl. dementia	59–102	378	92	24.3
Brandon et al.	1971	Mixed, incl. dementia	51–80 +	259	86	33.2
Delwaide and Desseiles	1977	Mixed, no dementia	60–99	55	16	29.1
		Mixed, incl. dementia	60–99	185	72	38.9

been compared in the same study in patients who were and were not exposed to neuroleptics, prevalences were higher in the neuroleptic-treated group (36, 35); this agrees with the age-corrected study of Owens and his colleagues (8, 29). The earlier study of Brandon et al. (27) superficially showed no overall excess of abnormal movements in patients who have received neuroleptics over those who have not. However, careful reappraisal of these data reveals that such movements were significantly more prevalent in neuroleptic-treated patients over age 50, and that a substantial majority of the group showing abnormal movements in the absence of neuroleptic exposure showed clinical signs of dementia (4, 5, 39).

It may be that the phenomenon of abnormal movements in patients not exposed to neuroleptics is a manifestation of (sometimes subtle) brain damage in psychotic disorders and classical organic brain disease. Neuroleptics may enhance such processes, elevating to a varying extent the baseline prevalence of abnormal movements (32). The extent to which those 'irreversible' movements persisting after neuroleptic withdrawal have their basis in disease rather than neuroleptic-related processes appears to have been underestimated.

REFERENCES

1. Klawans HL, Goetz CG, Perlik S: Tardive dyskinesia: review and update. Am J Psychiatry 137:900–908, 1980

2. Jeste DV, Wyatt RJ: Changing epidemiology of tardive dyskinesia: an overview. Am J Psychiatry 138:297–309, 1981

3. Jeste DV, Wyatt RJ: Therapeutic strategies against tardive dyskinesia. Arch Gen Psychiatry 39:803–816, 1982

4. Kane JM, Smith JM: Tardive dyskinesia: prevalence and risk factors, 1959 to 1979. Arch Gen Psychiatry 39:473–481, 1982

5. Waddington JL: Tardive dyskinesia: a critical evaluation of the causal role of neuroleptics and the dopamine receptor supersensitivity hypothesis, in Recent Research in Neurology. Edited by Callaghan N, Galvin R. London, Pitman, 1984, pp. 34–48

6. Yarden PE, DiScipio WJ: Abnormal movements and prognosis in schizophrenia. Am J Psychiatry 128:317–323, 1971

7. Stevens J: Motor disorders in schizophrenia. N Engl J Med 290:110, 1974

8. Owens DGC, Johnstone EC, Frith CD: Spontaneous involuntary disorders of movement, their prevalence, severity and distribution in chronic schizophrenics with and without treatment with neuroleptics. Arch Gen Psychiatry 39:452–461, 1982

9. Diller T: Chorea in the adult as seen among the insane. Am J Med Sci 99:329–349, 1980

10. Kraepelin E: Dementia Praecox and Paraphrenia. Translated by Barclay RM. New York, Krieger, 1971 (original 1919)

11. Bleuler E: Dementia Praecox or the Group of Schizophrenias (1911). Translated by Zinkin J. New York, International Universities Press, 1950

12. Farran-Ridge C: Some symptoms referrable to the basal ganglia occurring in dementia praecox and epidemic encephalitis. J Ment Sci 72:513–523, 1926

13. Reiter PJ: Extrapyramidal motor disturbances in dementia praecox. Acta Psychiatr Neurol 1:287–305, 1926

14. Jelliffe SE: The mental pictures in schizophrenia and in epidemic encephalitis, in Schizophrenia. Edited by Dana CL. New York, P.B. Hoeber, 1928

15. Jones MR: Measurement of spontaneous movements in adult psychotic patients by a time-sample technique: a methodological study. J Psychol 11:285–295, 1941

16. Leonhard K: Die Defektschizophrenen Krankheitsbilder. Leipzig, Georg Thieme, 1936

17. Leonhard K: Aufteilung der Endogenen Psychosen. Berlin, Akadamie-Verlag 1957. Translated into English as "The Classification of Endogenous Psychoses." New York, Irvington, 1979

18. Fish F: Leonhard's classification of schizophrenia. J Ment Sci 104:943–971, 1958

19. Fish F: The influence of tranquillizers on the Leonhard schizophrenic syndromes. Encephale 1:245–249, 1964

20. Tarsy D, Baldessarini RJ: The tardive dyskinesia syndrome. Clin Neuropharmacol 1:29–61, 1976

21. Simpson GM, Lee JH, Zoubok B: A rating scale for tardive dyskinesia. Psychopharmacology 64:171–179, 1979

22. Kucharski LT, Smith JM, Dunn DD: Tardive dyskinesia and hospital discharge. J Nerv Ment Dis 168:215–218, 1980

23. Chouinard G, Annable L, Ross-Chouinard A, et al: Factors related to tardive dyskinesia. Am J Psychiatry 136:79–83, 1979

24. Smith JM, Baldessarini RJ: Changes in prevalence, severity and recovery in tardive dyskinesia with age. Arch Gen Psychiatry 37:1368–1373, 1980

25. Klawans HL, Barr A: Prevalence of spontaneous lingual–facial–buccal dyskinesias in the elderly. Neurology 32:558–559, 1982

26. Kane JM, Weinhold P, Kinon B, et al: Prevalence of abnormal involuntary movements ("spontaneous dyskinesias") in the normal elderly. Psychopharmacology 77:105–108, 1982

27. Brandon S, McClelland HA, Protheroe C: A study of facial dyskinesia in a mental hospital population. Br J Psychiatry 118:171–184, 1971

28. Waddington JL, Youssef HA, O'Boyle KM, et al: A reappraisal of abnormal, involuntary movements ("tardive dyskinesia") in schizophrenia and other disorders, in The Neurobiology of Dopamine Systems. Edited by Winlow W, Markstein R. Manchester, Manchester Univ Press, 1986, pp. 266–286

29. Crow TJ, Owens DGC, Johnstone EC, et al: Does tardive dyskinesia exist? Mod Probl Pharmacopsychiatry 21:206–219, 1983

30. Crow TJ: Molecular pathology of schizophrenia: more than one disease process? Br Med J 280:66–68, 1980

31. Crow TJ: The two syndrome concept: origins and current status. Schizophr Bull 11:471–486, 1985

32. Waddington JL: Tardive dyskinesia in schizophrenia and other disorders: associations with aging, cognitive dysfunction and structural brain pathology in relation to neuroleptic exposure. Human Psychopharmacology 2:11–22, 1987

33. Martinelli P, Gabellini AS: Essential tremor and buccolinguofacial dyskinesias. Acta Neurol Scand 66:705–798, 1982

34. Delwaide PJ, Desseiles M: Spontaneous buccolinguofacial dyskinesia in the elderly. Acta Neurol Scand 56:256–262, 1977

35. Blowers AJ: Epidemiology of tardive dyskinesia in the elderly. Neuropharmacology 20:1339–1340, 1981

36. Bourgeois M, Bouilh P, Tignol J, et al: Spontaneous dyskinesias vs neuroleptic induced dyskinesias in 270 elderly subjects. J Nerv Ment Dis 168:177–178, 1980

37. Molsa PK, Martilla RJ, Rinne UK: Extrapyramidal symptoms in dementia. Acta Neurol Scand 65 (Suppl 90):298–299, 1982

38. Molsa PK, Martilla RJ, Rinne UK: Extrapyramidal signs in Alzheimer's disease. Neurology 34:1114–1116, 1984

39. Toenniessen LM, Casey DE, McFarland BH: Tardive dyskinesia in the aged: duration of treatment relationships. Arch Gen Psychiatry 42:278–284, 1985

Chapter 6

Tardive Dyskinesia: Clinical Features

Hardeep Singh, M.D.
George M. Simpson, M.D.

Chapter 6

Tardive Dyskinesia:
Clinical Features

The introduction of neuroleptic agents in the early 1950s ushered in a period of therapeutic optimism. It had a profound effect on psychiatric practice and stimulated much biomedical research. Soon after, abnormal movements—later named tardive dyskinesia (TD)—were observed in patients taking neuroleptics. This chapter reviews recent research on definition, diagnosis, clinical signs, and the factors that increase risk of TD.

HISTORICAL ASPECTS

Schonecker (1) reported four patients who developed "a peculiar syndrome in the oral region as a result of Megaphen (chlorpromazine)" (pp. 28–35). Sigwald et al. (2) described four patients with chronic dyskinesia that persisted for months after neuroleptics were discontinued. Sigwald, a careful observer, believed that although these dyskinesias were neuroleptic induced, the type and dose of neuroleptic were not important in the etiology of TD. He believed that the dyskinesias would probably disappear slowly over a period of time.

A number of cases of reversible dyskinesia were described between 1957 and 1959. Uhrbrand and Faurbye (3) observed two cases of irreversible buccolingual masticatory dyskinesia. The authors observed that these two cases arose after electroconvulsive therapy and were presumed to be due to some organic lesion. These investigators also reported 29 cases of dyskinetic syndrome consisting of involuntary grimaces, mastication, and propulsion of the tongue (3). They observed that these movements had developed in neuroleptic-treated patients. Fifteen cases had been treated with perphenazine, ten cases with chlorpromazine, one case with reserpine and three cases with various compounds. This dyskinesia was described as occurring late in the treatment period and was thus called tardive dyskinesia, in contrast to reversible dyskinetic symptoms, which occurred at an early stage of the treatment. The authors concluded from their observations that prolonged administration of psychopharmacological agents, which cause neurological side effects, carries the risk of lesions on the central nervous system (CNS) with irreversible dyskinesias, especially in elderly patients and patients with organic brain diseases.

Kruse (4) described three patients who had developed persistent muscular restlessness after treatment with high doses of phenothiazines. The three patients were 50 years or older. In all three cases, the feeling of subjective restlessness was accompanied by occasional jerky, involuntary movements of the limbs. One patient had also developed involuntary lip and tongue movements. The signs and symptoms persisted for 3 to 18 months after the drugs were stopped. This led Kruse to question whether phenothiazines were always as innocuous as people believed them to be.

DEFINITION OF TARDIVE DYSKINESIA

Since 1960, hundreds of papers have been written on TD, and this research has played a large and, as yet, incomplete role in changing the concept of TD. Recent research has focused on providing a more critical definition of the syndrome. Originally, abnormal movements of the face, mouth and tongue, the so-called buccolingual masticatory syndromes, were considered the defining symptoms of TD. Now, choreoathetoid movements of the hands, feet, and arms and respiratory dyskinesia are also included (5).

A variety of standardized measuring devices developed for use in prospective studies, clinical trails, and epidemiological surveys helped advance the evaluation and understanding of TD (6, 7). Much effort has gone into distinguishing withdrawal TD from persistent TD (8, 9). From the earliest use of neuroleptics, it has been known that TD often appears after a neuroleptic has been withdrawn and that in many of these cases, the condition improves or disappears (10–12). The rate of disappearance of withdrawal dyskinesia has been quoted as anywhere from 0 to 90 percent (13). This wide disparity suggests that different populations were studied, or at the very least, different methodologies were used.

Suffice it to say that if we were to abruptly withdraw neuroleptics from a large number of subjects, a large percentage would develop a dyskinesia, particularly if they had been on high dosages. In a substantial number of these subjects, dyskinesia would disappear in weeks or in months at most. Persistent TD occurs when dyskinetic movements persist for more than 3 months after withdrawal of neuroleptics. Many investigators comment that this is too short a time period. Data do exist to show that persistent dyskinesia improves long after 3 months, that is, even persistent dyskinesia is not irreversible.

Research Diagnostic Criteria have been developed to clarify withdrawal and persistent TD (14). The three prerequisites are as follows:

1. A history of at least 3 months total cumulative neuroleptic exposure. Exposure may be continuous or discontinuous. Patients who fail to meet the criterion or duration of neuroleptic exposure would receive the appropriate diagnosis with the qualification "less than 3 months neuroleptic exposure." Include all of the following classes of neuroleptics: phenothiazines (for example, chlorpromazine hydrochloride), substituted benzamines (for example, sulpiride), dibenzoxazepines (for example, loxapine), dihydroindolones (for example, molindone), and diphenylbutylpiperidines (for example, penfluridol).
2. The presence of at least "moderate" abnormal, involuntary movements in one or more body areas or at least "mild" movements in two or more body areas (face, lips, jaw, tongue, upper extremities, lower extremities, or trunk). Because of the variability in the manifestation of movements associated with TD, if the examination reveals movements that are only "minimal" or "mild" in only one body area, the examination should be repeated within 1 week to confirm their presence. Determination of the presence of these movements should be made using a standardized examination procedure and rating scale (e.g., the Abnormal Involuntary Movement Scale or the Rockland Simpson Tardive Dyskinesia Scale).
3. Absence of other conditions that might produce abnormal involuntary movements.

These prerequisites and the following diagnostic classification do not allow us to distinguish between TD and stereotyped movements of schizophrenia, spontaneous oral dyskinesias of advanced age or senility, and oral dyskinesia related to dental conditions or prostheses. However, it is hoped that the careful application of these criteria to various populations may provide us with the ability to separate these phenomena.

DIAGNOSES

As should become clear on reading the definitions that follow, the diagnoses are "progressive." On first evaluation, the only TD diagnosis possible is probably TD. It is not until a subsequent evaluation that any other TD diagnosis is possible. At a second or later evaluation, it is necessary to determine 1) whether movements have remained the same, appeared, or disappeared; 2) whether neuroleptic dosage has changed; and 3) over what length of time movements and medication have or have not been present. With knowledge of these factors, the diagnoses, whose definitions follow, can be assigned.

1. Probably TD—The patient meets the three prerequisites. The diagnosis is qualified as either "concurrent neuroleptics" if the patient is currently receiving neuroleptics or "neuroleptic free" if the patient is not currently receiving neuroleptics.
2. Masked probably TD—The patient meets the criteria for probably TD but within 2 weeks, following an increase in dosage (in the case of concurrent neuroleptics) or reinstitution of neuroleptic treatment (in the case of a neuroleptic-free patient), movements no longer meet prerequisite 2.
3. Transient TD—The patient meets the criteria for probably TD, but on subsequent examination within 3 months the movements meeting prerequisite 2 no longer are observed and neuroleptic treatment has not been reinstituted (for the neuroleptic-free patient) or the dosage has not been increased (for patients receiving concurrent neuroleptic treatment). (Downward dosage adjustments may have occurred.)
4. Withdrawal TD—The patient does not meet prerequisite 2 (that is, severity of movements) while receiving neuroleptics, but does so within 2 weeks following neuroleptic discontinuation (5 weeks for "long-acting drugs," such as fluphenazine decanoate or penfluridol). If within 3 months of drug withdrawal, the movements meeting prerequisite 2 are no longer observed, the diagnosis stands.
5. Persistent TD—The patient meets the criteria for probably TD and continues to do so over a 3-month period. The diagnosis may be qualified as "concurrent neuroleptics" if the patient has been receiving neuroleptics continuously during the 3-month period; as "neuroleptic free" if the patient has received no neuroleptics during the 3-month period or has met the criteria for withdrawal TD, but the movements meeting prerequisite 2 have persisted for at least 3 months with no neuroleptic administration; or as "unspecified" if the patient has received neuroleptics for part but not all of the 3-month period.
6. Masked persistent TD—The patient meeting the criteria for persistent TD but within 3 weeks following the increase in dosage (for patients receiving neuroleptics) or reinstitution of neuroleptic

treatment (for neuroleptic-free patients) the movements no longer meet prerequisite 2.

CLINICAL DESCRIPTION

TD has been described many times in many ways. All descriptions share an emphasis on the presence of buccolingual masticatory movements and choreoathetoid movements of the limbs, especially their distal portions and movements of the trunk and neck. Most descriptions exclude obvious parkinsonian tremor of the extremities, although tremors of the upper lip, rabbit syndrome, tongue and eyelids are sometimes included in descriptions of TD. We would now not agree with their inclusion. Restless movements of the legs (akathisia) frequently occur along with the more typical dyskinetic movements of TD. Complex, semipurposeful mannerisms are usually excluded from the syndrome where these appear to be manifestations of the patients' psychoses.

It is important to emphasize that TD movements are irregular, and therefore regular, rhythmical movements are not TD. The early description of this syndrome stressed abnormal motor movements affecting the face, the so-called buccolingual masticatory syndrome. This consisted of involuntary mouthing movements, chewing, and smacking movements of the lips associated with abnormal movements of the tongue, which frequently darted from the oral cavity, and thus was referred to as fly-catcher's tongue. Later, this syndrome was broadened to include a variety of abnormal muscular manifestations, for example, choreoathetoid type movements of the fingers, hands, arms, and feet; ballistic-type movements, particularly of the arms; axial hyperkinesis; and diaphragmatic involvement resulting in grunting and difficult breathing.

Some signs are complex enough to make description and quantification difficult, for example, abnormal or neurological gait seen in association with severe dyskinesia. These gaits range from a stamping-type gait to a broad-base or sailor gait with other, even more complex, gaits. There are also certain unusual movements seen in individual patients (diaphragmatic spasms, irregular speech patterns, complex object touching). All these movements or gaits can be considered a part of the TD syndrome.

Description of Some Common Movements Seen as a Part of TD

1. Pouting of lower lip. A thrusting out of the lower lip as in solemnness.
2. Puckering of lips. Drawstring or pursing action of the lips.

3. Smacking of lips. Brisk separation of lips that produces a sharp sound.
4. Sucking movements.
5. Chewing movements.
6. Bon-bon sign. Tongue movements within the oral cavity which produces a bulge in the cheek giving the impression that the patient has a hard "bon-bon" candy pocketed in cheek. Occasionally, a repetitious, sweeping movement with tongue over the buccal lining, which also pushes out of the mouth.
7. Tongue protrusion. Clonic, arrhythmic, in and out movements of the tongue. Tonic and continuous protrusion of the tongue. Fly-catcher—a sudden shooting out of the tongue from the mouth at irregular episodes.
8. Choreoathetoid movements of the tongue. A rolling, worm-like movement of the tongue muscles without displacement of the tongue from the mouth. The tongue may rotate on its longitudinal axis. Observed when the mouth is open and the tongue is within the buccal cavity.
9. Facial tics. Brief, recurrent stereotyped movement involving the relatively small segments of the face.
10. Grimacing. A repetitive, irregular-occurring distortion of the face. A complex movement involving large segments of facial muscles.
11. Head nodding. Slower than tremor, may or may not be rhythmic. Can occur horizontally or vertically.*
12. Axial hyperkinesia. A front-to-back hip-rocking movement. Resembles copulatory movements. Differs from the rocking movement, in which it is the upper torso which has to-and-fro movement.*
13. Rocking movements. A rhythmic, to-and-fro movement of the upper torso that occurs from a repeated bending of the spinal column in the lumbar region. Different from axial hyperkinesia where the hips move to and fro.*
14. Ballistic movements. Sudden, fast, large-amplitude swinging movements occurring most often in the arms and less frequently in the legs. One or both sides may be involved.
15. Choreiform movements. In fingers, wrists, arms. Variable, purposeless, course, quick jerky movements that begin suddenly and show no rhythmicity. They vary in distribution and extension.
16. Athetoid movements. In fingers, wrists, arms. Continuous

---

*These may seem contradictory to our earlier statement that TD is regular and nonrhythmical, but clinically we have observed this frequently enough to include it with TD.

rhythmic, slow writing, worm-like movements. They almost invariably appear together with choreiform movements.
17. Finger counting. Rhythmic rubbing of the thumb against the middle and index fingers.*
18. Caressing face and hair. Gives the impression of an absent-minded or nervous mannerism; has the appearance of being purposeful.
19. Rubbing of thighs. Hands rub the outside or top of thighs. Sporadic and nonrhythmic.
20. Rotation and/or flexion of the ankles.
21. Toe movements. Slow, rhythmic retroflexion, usually of the big toes although other toes can also be involved.
22. Stamping movements (standing). Weight is shifted back and forth from one foot to the other when patient stands.†
23. Stamping movements (sitting). Flapping or tapping of whole foot on floor or may take the form of an alternate toe and heel tapping.†
24. Akathisia or restless legs. Constant leg movement, jiggling of toes or foot when leg is crossed. May involve rapidly moving knees apart and together. An inability to sit or stand still (the verbal expression of inner restlessness is not required here).†
25. Crossing and uncrossing of legs.
26. Holokinetic movements. Extensive, jerky, rapid, abrupt, awkward, gross movements of large parts of or the entire body. The movement may appear to be somewhat goal directed and only moderately coordinated. May begin in response to stimulus or spontaneous.

DIFFERENTIAL DIAGNOSIS

Much information about the differential diagnosis of TD has accrued, but a simple, pathological sign for TD has yet to be identified. There is new evidence that oral dyskinesia, a common symptom of TD, may occur in drug-free elderly populations at a rate higher than the early estimate of 2 percent (15). One study estimated the incidence of oral dyskinesia in a nursing home population never treated with neuroleptics to be as high as 37 percent (16). A more recent finding suggests that 4 percent is a reasonable figure for elderly subjects never treated with neuroleptics.

At the same time, there are reports that nonneuroleptic drugs

---

*These may seem contradictory to our earlier statement that TD is regular and nonrhythmical, but clinically we have observed this frequently enough to include it with TD.

†These may resemble and/or be part of akathisia.

(including antihistamines, phenytoin, and tricyclic antidepressants) are, on rare occasions, associated with TD (17–19).

Other disorders such as stereotyped movements of schizophrenia, Gilles de la Tourette syndrome, Wilson's disease, atypical torsion dystonias, and Huntington's chorea can be confused with TD (18). The cognitive changes in Huntington's chorea and Wilson's disease along with lab findings, computerized tomographic scan results, and family history help to differentiate these conditions from tardive dyskinesia. Distinguishing TD from some of these progressively degenerative conditions is TD's stability over time. After the onset of TD, there is a reasonably long period during which symptoms do not change. Indeed, studies have shown that even with continued neuroleptic use, tardive dyskinesia may decrease over time. Assessment of the patient's history and the characteristic features and progression of the condition help the clinician make a differential diagnosis.

We consider that tardive dystonia is a much rarer disorder than TD that affects young adults after only brief exposure to neuroleptics. It tends to affect the neck muscles first and presents as opisthotonos or abnormal head position. To that extent, it is similar to the acute dystonic reactions that patients may develop in the first few days of neuroleptic treatment. However, tardive dystonia is a persistent disorder that usually does not disappear when neuroleptics are withdrawn.

We have observed that abnormal tongue movements are absent early in the course of tardive dystonia, but they can develop later in a small number of cases, perhaps in association with the high doses of anticholinergics that are used to treat the condition. The spasm of the neck muscles in tardive dystonia is prolonged and may extend to muscles of the shoulder girdle and, ultimately, the trunk. In extreme cases, the subject's head may be continuously retracted so that walking is virtually impossible and from direct frontal view the subject's face and eyes are not visible. Such patients rest their heads against solid objects in an attempt to relieve the spasm and may walk in close contact with a wall. Movements may interfere with the patient's eating. Hemiballistic arm movement may occur, but the patient may be able to modify them so they appear purposeful.

There is no definite treatment for tardive dystonia. High doses of anticholinergics are claimed to be of benefit (20), but some patients do not respond to them (21). Trials of baclofen and high doses of benzodiazepines, such as clonazepam, have been attempted with varying degrees of success. If severe, restarting of neuroleptics may be required. In extreme cases, surgical intervention may be necessary (22). Some cases of tardive dystonia may represent late-onset congenital torsion dystonias that were provoked or unmasked by neuroleptics. In those cases, treatment would be the same as for torsion dystonias.

PREDISPOSING FACTORS

Increasing age is the most consistent risk factor for TD (23, 24). This finding has yet to be explained but may be related to pathological changes in the brain associated with the aging process, which have also been demonstrated in animals (25).

There is a higher prevalence of TD among women, mainly in upper age groups. The reason for this difference is unclear (26). It has been postulated that estrogen, which modulates dopamine receptor sensitivity, may protect young women from TD (26, 27).

Except for age and sex, factors that increase vulnerability to TD remain uncertain (28–31). However, the reports of TD in young adults following brief exposure to neuroleptics (11) and an early onset of severely debilitating TD in children and adolescents taking neuroleptics (32) indicate that individual susceptibility must play a large role in the development of TD.

Several studies have suggested that higher doses of neuroleptics may be related to higher prevalence and severity of TD (29, 33–35). Other studies, including a transcultural study, have not confirmed that correlation (28, 31, 36, 37). Kane and Smith reviewed 56 reports of TD prevalence and risk factors and found 18 studies that explored the relationship between cumulative drug dose and TD prevalence. Of these, 4 studies reported a significant positive relationship and 14 did not.

These positive studies generally focus on patients with relatively brief or low total dose exposure. Recently, a low prevalence and lack of severe forms of TD in patients who were treated with very low doses of depot fluphenazine were reported (38). Crane and Smeets reported significantly less TD in individuals who had received less than 12.6 g of chlorpromazine than in those who received more. Heinrich et al. (39) found a similar relationship using a total cumulative dose of 100 g of chlorpromazine equivalents as a cut-off, which would average 274 mg/day for 1 year. Crane (34) reported a higher prevalence of TD among patients treated with 80 mg/day of trifluoperazine compared to those receiving 16 mg/day over a 6-month period. Interpretation of these results is difficult, since the differences were not significant at the end of the actual trial; rather, significant differences emerged only after 6 months of additional follow-up. During this additional follow-up period, the patients who were getting a higher dose underwent a substantial dosage reduction, which may have resulted in unmasking covert or latent dyskinesias. On the other hand, the low-dose group continued to receive doses similar to those received during the initial 6 months, and the prevalence of abnormal movements remained essentially unchanged during the 6-month follow-up period. These data highlight the importance of identifying an appropriate endpoint to examine patients exposed to different dosages.

Kane et al. (40) have conducted two studies that provide an opportunity to examine the issue of dosage in relation to TD development and in relationship to the course of DT once it occurs.

The first study was a prospective, double-blind, random assignment comparison of two discrete dosage ranges of fluphenazine decanoate. The two dosage ranges were 12.5 to 50 mg and 1.25 to 5 mg given every other week. To determine the presence of abnormal involuntary movements, a modified version of the Rockland Simpson Tardive Dyskinesia Scale was used. For the purposes of this analysis, only patients who participated in the study for at least 24 weeks were included. The groups did not differ significantly at baseline. Despite the fact that the sample as a whole had very little dyskinetic symptomatology, a significant difference did emerge at end point, indicating an advantage for a low dose in producing fewer early signs of TD. The second study that provides data on the influence of neuroleptic dosage on the course of TD is a large-scale prospective study of TD development. Preliminary analysis on the course of TD was conducted in which data were analyzed from 98 patients who developed TD during the time they participated in the study. These patients had been followed for up to 7 years after their developing TD. On the basis of the entire follow-up course, each patient was classified as remitted, masked, or persistent. Analysis of outcome over 2 years of follow-up indicated that a total of 32 percent of the patients remitted over the first year, and a total of 47 percent of the patients remitted within the first 2 years. For each patient, the modal dose of neuroleptic taken during the follow-up period was estimated. Range of these modal doses was 0 to 2000 mg (in chlorpromazine equivalents). Further analysis of the data showed that the modal dose of neuroleptics following development of TD was a critical factor in the likelihood of remission, with patients treated with lower modal doses more likely to remit. For example, among patients receiving modal doses equivalent to 500 mg of chlorpromazine following TD development, 50 percent would show remission of TD within 120 weeks. It was also shown that remission was more likely for patients spending less time on medication. In addition, prognosis for remission was better for patients who developed TD following short exposure to neuroleptics than it was for patients who developed TD following long exposure. Thus, these authors have concluded the modal dose following TD is a critical variable, with an impact over and above the effect of prior medication history.

It has been suggested that neuroleptic drug holidays may increase the risk of developing TD. One retrospective study and review of this issue associated frequent drug holidays with high rates of irreversible TD (41). In contrast, when neuroleptics were discontinued at early signs of TD, but periodically represcribed during psychotic episodes, TD resolved or improved to a minimally present and stable level over 3 to 7 years (42). Carpenter et al. (43) have published a preliminary analysis from a continuous versus intermittent (targeted) drug study that supports the hypothesis that targeted medication is associated with reduced incidence of TD. Subjects were outpatients with a *Diagnostic and Statistical Manual of Mental Disorders (Third Edition* (44) diagnosis of schizophrenia who were randomly assigned to either continuous (55 patients) or targeted (41 patients) medication for a 2-year treatment course. Twenty-four new cases of TD were identified, 18 on continuous and 6 on targeted medication. The probability of a continuous drug patient developing abnormal movements was 2.83 times those of a targeted drug patient developing such symptoms. Within the targeted sample, those patients who developed TD were characterized by more days on medication and higher cumulative dose than the remainder of the group. Gardos and Cole (45) found neuroleptic-free periods to be characteristic of only mild cases of TD while severe TD cases were significantly more often treated continuously. In general, there are far too few data to adequately address the relative effects of interrupted versus continuous drug therapy in the outcome of TD, but one can feel optimistic about this strategy.

It has been proposed that some antipsychotic drugs have more of a propensity to produce TD than do other antipsychotic drugs. Virtually all available neuroleptics have been associated with TD. Efforts to identify classes of neuroleptics that pose a higher risk have produced inconclusive and confusing results. For instance, some authors (46, 47) have claimed depot forms of neuroleptics, such as fluphenazine decant, increase the risk of TD but others (48) have claimed depot forms are associated with a lower risk of TD than are oral neuroleptics. Low-potency neuroleptics have also been reported to pose a greater risk for TD. All of these data must be interpreted cautiously; none represent convincing evidence that any one neuroleptic is more or less likely to be associated with TD. Much of the evidence comes from weak associations and there are pitfalls in this type of retrospective epidemiological study. The drug administered last is likely to be put forward as the culprit, but to date there are no data showing differences between different drugs in the potential for causing TD.

Two studies (49, 50) found higher plasma levels of neuroleptics in patients with TD compared to those without TD, suggesting that TD patients do not metabolize neuroleptics as efficiently as patients who do not develop TD. Again, contradictory data was reported by other investigations (51).

The relationship of TD to another side effect of neuroleptic drugs, parkinsonism, and other drugs used to treat it has been carefully evaluated (52, 53). Several studies have described the coexistence of TD and parkinsonism (54–56). Recent data have lent renewed support to an early idea that the severity of patients' parkinsonism could predict whether the patient would develop TD (38), a concept that studies over the years have failed to confirm (57–60). Contrary to speculation, antiparkinson agents have not been shown to predispose patients to TD, although they may exacerbate or unmask it (61).

Increased awareness of TD plays a major role in the trend toward the higher rates being reported in recent years. Many problems have resulted from the widespread notion of TD being an "epidemic." Both TD and spontaneous dyskinesia prevalence increased at similar rates, suggesting that the "epidemic" of TD is more apparent than real. For example, criteria for diagnosis have changed so that a more balanced evaluation of the scope of the problem is possible, with increasing attention to the problem of TD and with the same attention paid to control groups, age, and size of the study plus methodological improvements. Unfortunately, studies with the ideal control group (drug-free schizophrenics) are lacking and it remains unclear whether schizophrenia itself is a risk factor for TD, as suggested by Owens et al. (62). Mentally retarded subjects treated with neuroleptics show similar age and sex predisposition to TD. It has also been claimed that patients suffering from affective disorders are at a greater risk for developing TD than are patients who have other psychiatric disorders (63–66). It is as yet questionable as to whether a particular diagnosis predicts who may or may not develop TD.

PATIENT VARIABLES THAT AFFECT THE OUTCOME OF TD

Age. Age is a factor most consistently correlated with outcome of TD. Younger patients are more likely to improve (24, 30, 41, 67, 68). However, this trend does not exclude or guarantee symptom resolution in any group, since TD in some elderly patients improves over several years. Similarly, there are some young patients who develop TD that persists. Overall, the relationship between age and the onset and/or persistence of TD is similar. The elderly are at a higher risk for developing TD and are less likely to have it resolved. *Sex.* Most but not all studies report that TD is more likely to develop in women.

Psychiatric Diagnosis. Few comparative data exist about the long-term outcome of TD in patients with different psychiatric diagnosis. The use of neuroleptics in a nonschizophrenic population is somewhat controversial. It is also clear that neuroleptics are useful in several nonschizophrenic conditions. However, these conditions themselves may be risk factors for the development of TD, and this indeed is a considerable problem.

Time Period. It is necessary to evaluate over a long period of time TD patients whose past and present drug treatments can be quantified. Without these multiple assessments, information can be misleading. For example, TD may initially appear when drug dosage is reduced because symptoms are unmasked. These unmasked symptoms may gradually improve; however, this may be an important observation that may be missed without long-term follow-up. Similarly, TD symptoms may decrease when drug dosage is increased, because symptoms are masked or suppressed.

The majority of data suggest that discontinuing neuroleptic drugs leads to stabilization or gradual improvement of symptoms. There is considerably less information about the outcome of TD when neuroleptics must be continued. The overall finding is that TD does not inevitably worsen with continued neuroleptic treatment. This does mean that TD cannot get worse. Nonetheless, low to moderate doses (300 to 600 mg/day of chlorpromazine equivalents) are also associated with a course of stabilizing or improving TD symptoms. These findings clearly demonstrate that TD is not inevitably aggravated with continued neuroleptic treatment.

CONCLUSION

Tardive dyskinesia remains a perplexing problem for clinicians and for patients and their families. Considerable research is being conducted to identify new risk factors. Elderly females are at most risk, and there is evidence that higher dosages of neuroleptics may also be a risk factor. All neuroleptics appear equally likely to suppress the symptoms of schizophrenia and to cause TD. Therefore care should be taken to prescribe neuroleptics only to patients for whom no other treatment is effective. Clinicians should attempt to reduce the dosage required to treat acute episodes early in treatment. They should also carefully monitor for signs of TD and attempt to reduce or even withdraw the neuroleptics.

REFERENCES

1. Schonecker M: Ein eigentumliches Syndrom in eralen Bereich bei. Megaphen Applikation Nervenarzt 28:35, 1957

2. Sigwald J, Bouttier D, Raymondeand C, et al: Quatre cas de dyskinesie facio-bucco-lingui-masticatrice a evolution prolongee secondaire a un traitment par les neuroleptiques. Revue Neurologique 100:751–755, 1959

3. Uhrbrand L, Faurbye A: Reversible and irreversible dyskinesia after treatment with perphernazine, chlorpromazine, reserpine, and electroconvulsive therapy. Psychopharmacologia 1:408–418, 1960

4. Kruse W: Persistent muscular restlessness after phenothiazine treatment: report of 3 cases. Am J Psychiatry 117:152–153, 1960

5. Simpson GM, Pi EH, Sramek JJ: Adverse effects of antipsychotic agents. Drugs 21:138–151, 1981

6. Guy W (ed): ECDEU Assessment Manual for Psychopharmacology (U.S. Department of Health, Education and Welfare Publication 76-338). Washington, DC, U.S. Government Printing Office, 1976

7. Simpson GM, Lee JH, Zoubok B, et al: A rating scale for tardive dyskinesia. Psychopharmacology 64:171–179, 1979

8. Kennedy PF, Herschen HL, McGuire RJ: Extrapyramidal disorders after prolonged phenothiazine therapy. Br J Psychiatry 118:509–518, 1971

9. Kazamatsuri H, Chien CP, Cole JO: Treatment of tardive dyskinesia, II: Short-term efficacy of dopamine-blocking agents, haloperidol and thiopropazate. Arch Gen Psychiatry 27:100–103, 1982

10. Crane GE: Rapid reversal of tardive dyskinesia. Am J Psychiatry 130:1159, 1973

11. Simpson GM: Tardive dyskinesia. Br J Psychiatry 122:618, 1973

12. Moline RA: Atypical tardive dyskinesia. Am J Psychiatry 132:534–535, 1975

13. American College of Neuropsychopharmacology–Food and Drug Administration Task Force: Neurological syndromes associated with antipsychotic drug use. Arch Gen Psychiatry 28:463–466, 1973

14. Schooler NR, Kane JM: Research diagnoses for tardive dyskinesia. Arch Gen Psychiatry 39:486–487, 1982

15. Varga E, Sugarman AA, Varge V, et al: Prevalence of spontaneous oral dyskinesia in the elderly. Am J Psychiatry 139:329–331, 1982

16. Delwaide PJ, Desseilles M: Spontaneous buccolingual facial dyskinesia in the elderly. Acta Neurol Scand 56:256–262, 1977

17. Chadwick D, Reynolds EH, Marsden CD: Anticonvulsant-induced dyskinesia. A comparison with dyskinesias induced by neuroleptics. J Neurol 39:120–121, 1976

18. David WA: Dyskinesia associated with chronic antihistamine use. N Engl J Med 194:113, 1976

19. Fann W, Sullivan JL, Richman B: Dyskinesias associated with tricyclic antidepressants. Br J Psychiatry 128:490–493, 1976

20. Fahn S: Treatment of tardive dyskinesia, use of dopamine depleting agents. Clin Neuropharmacol 6:151–158, 1983

21. Wolf ME, Koller WC: Tardive dystonia: treatment with trihexiphenidyl. J Clin Psychopharmacol 5:247–248, 1985

22. Goldman HW, Cooper IS, Simpson GM, et al: Reversal of tardive dyskinesia and dystonia following bilateral CT-guided stereotactic thalamotomy. Presented at the Fourth World Congress on Biologic Psychiatry, Philadelphia, PA, 1985

23. Smith JM, Kucharski LT, Eblen C, et al: An assessment of tardive dyskinesia in schizophrenic outpatients. Psychopharmacology 64:99–104, 1979

24. Smith JM, Baldessarini RJ: Changes in prevalence, severity and recovery in tardive dyskinesia with age. Arch Gen Psychiatry 37:1368–1373, 1980

25. Campbell A, Baldessarini RJ: Effects of maturation and aging on behavior responses to haloperidol in the rat. Psychopharmacology 73:219–222, 1981

26. Gordon J, Borison R, Diamond B: Modulation of dopamine receptor sensitivity by estrogen. Biol Psychiatry 15:389–396, 1980

27. Chouinard G, Jones B, Annable L, et al: Sex differences and tardive dyskinesia. Am J Psychiatry 137:507, 1980

28. Simpson GM, Varga E, Lee JH, et al: Tardive dyskinesia and psychotropic drug history. Psychopharmacology 58:117–124, 1978

29. Smith HM, Oswald WD, Kucharski T, et al: Tardive dyskinesia: age and sex differences in hospitalized schizophrenics. Psychopharmacology 58:207–211, 1978

30. Yassa R, Nair V: Incidence of tardive dyskinesia in an outpatient population. Psychosomatics 25:479–481, 1984

31. Baldessarini RJ: Clinical and epidemiologic aspects of tardive dyskinesia. J Clin Psychiatry 46:8–13, 1985

32. Gualtieri CT, Quade D, Hicks RE, et al: Tardive dyskinesia and other clinical consequences of neuroleptic treatment in children and adolescents. Am J Psychiatry 141:20–23, 1984

33. Pryce IG, Edward H: Persistent oral dyskinesia in female mental hospital patients. Br J Psychiatry 112:987, 1966

34. Crane GE: High doses of trifluoperazine and tardive dyskinesia. Arch Neurol 22:176–180, 1970

35. Crane GE, Smeets RA: Tardive dyskinesia and drug therapy in geriatric patients. Br J Psychiatry 30:341–343, 1976

36. Ojita K, Yogi G, Itoh H: Comparative analysis of persistent dyskinesia of long-term usage with neuroleptics in France and in Japan. Folia Psychiatrica et Neurologica 29:315–320, 1975

37. Kane JM, Smith JM: TD: prevalence and risk factors, 1959–1979. Arch Gen Psychiatry 39:473–481, 1982

38. Kane JM, Rifkin A, Woener M, et al: Low-dose neuroleptic treatment of outpatient schizophrenics. Arch Gen Psychiatry 40:893–896, 1983

39. Heinrich K, Wegener I, Bender HJ: Spate extrapyramidale hyperkinesen bei neuroleptischer lanzzeit-therapie. Pharmakopsychiatr Neuropsychopharmakol 1:169–195, 1968

40. Kane JM, Woerner M, Weinhold P, et al: Incidence and severity of tardive dyskinesia in affective illness, in Tardive Dyskinesia and Neuroleptics: From Dogma to Reason. Edited by Casey D, Gardos G. Washington, DC, American Psychiatric Press, 1986, pp.22–28

41. Jeste DV, Potkin SG, Linha S, et al: TD: reversible and persistent. Arch Gen Psychiatry 36:585–590, 1979

42. Wegner JT, Kane JM: Follow-up study on the reversibility of tardive dyskinesia. Am J Psychiatry 139:368–369, 1982

43. Carpenter WT, et al: Incidence of TD with intermittent pharmacotherapy. Paper presented at the 140th Annual Meeting of the American Psychiatric Association, Chicago, IL. May 1987

44. American Psychiatric Association: Diagnostic and Statistical Manual of Mental Disorders (Third Edition). Washington, DC, American Psychiatric Association, 1980

45. Gardos G, Cole JO: Early dyskinesia: course, outcome, and prognosis. Paper presented at the 135th Annual Meeting of the American Psychiatric Association, Toronto, Canada, May 1982

46. Gee S, Mesard L: Psychiatric Drug Study, Part I. Psychiatric Ward Unit Study (Office of the Controllers Monograph No. 9). Washington, DC, U.S. Veterans Administration, 1979

47. Csernansky JG, Grabowski K, Cervantes J, et al: Fluphenazine decanoate and TD: a possible association. Am J Psychiatry 138:1362–1365, 1981

48. Goldberg SC, Sheroy RS, Julius D, et al: Does long acting injectable neuroleptic protect against TD? Psychopharmacol Bull 18:177–179, 1982

49. Jeste DV, Rosenblatt JR, Wagner RL, et al: High serum levels in TD. N Engl J Med 301:1184, 1979

50. Perris C, Dimitrijevic P, Jacobsson L, et al: TD in psychiatric patients treated with neuroleptics. Br J Psychiatry 135:509–514, 1979

51. Fairbairn AF, Rowell FJ, Hui SM, et al: Serum concentration of depot neuroleptics in TD. Br J Psychiatry 142:579–583, 1983

52. Crane GE: Pseudoparkinsonism and TD. Arch Neurol 27:426–430, 1972

53. Gerlach J: The relationship between parkinsonism and TD. Am J Psychiatry 134:781–784, 1977

54. Chouinard G, Annable L, Ross-Chouinard A, et al: Ethopropazine and benztropine in neuroleptic-induced parkinsonism. J Clin Psychiatry 41:147–152, 1959

55. Fann WE, Lake CR: On the coexistence of parkinsonism and TD. Dis Nerv Syst 35:325–326, 1974

56. Defraites EG Jr, Davis KL, Berger PA: Coexisting TD and parkinsonism: a case report. Biol Psychiatry 12:147–152, 1977

57. Turek I, Kurland AA, Hanion TE, et al: TD: its relationship to neuroleptic and antiparkinson drugs. Br J Psychiatry 121:605–612, 1972

58. Kiloh IG, Smith SJ, Williams SE: Antiparkinson drugs as causal agents in TD. Med J Aust 2:591–593, 1973

59. Chouinard G, DeMontigny C, Annable L: TD and antiparkinsonian medication. Am J Psychiatry 136:228–229, 1979

60. Mukherjee S, Rosen AM, Cardenas C, et al: TD in psychiatric outpatients: a study of prevalence and association with demographic, clinical, and drug history variables. Arch Gen Psychiatry 39: 466–469, 1982

61. Gardos G, Cole JO: TD and anticholinergic drugs. Am J Psychiatry 140:200–202, 1983

62. Owen DGC, Johnstone EC, Frith CD: Spontaneous involuntary disorders of movement. Arch Gen Psychiatry 39:452–461, 1982

63. Yassa R, Ghadirian AM, Schwartz G: Prevalence of tardive dyskinesia in affective disorder patients. J Clin Psychiatry 44:410–412, 1983

64. Casey DE, Gerlach J: Tardive dyskinesia: management and new treatment, in Guidelines for the Use of Psychotropic Drugs. Edited by Stancer HC, Garfinkel PE, Rokoff VM. New York, SP Medical and Scientific Books, 1984

65. Wolf ME, DeWolfe AS, Ryan JJ, et al: Vulnerability to tardive dyskinesia. J Clin Psychitry 46:367–368, 1985

66. Kane JM, Woerner M, Wegner J, et al: Integration incidence and prevalence of TD. Psychopharmacol Bull 22:254–258, 1986

67. Seeman MV: TD: 2 year recovery. Compr Psychiatry 22:180–192, 1981

68. Smith JM, Burke MP, Moon CO: Long-term changes in AIMS rating and their relation to medication therapy. Psychopharmacol Bull 17:120–121, 1981

Chapter 7

Clinical Changes in Tardive Dyskinesia During Long-Term Follow-Up

Joseph DeVeaugh-Geiss, M.D.

Chapter 7

Clinical Changes in Tardive Dyskinesia During Long-Term Follow-Up

The syndrome of tardive dyskinesia (TD), an involuntary movement disorder associated with chronic use of neuroleptic (antipsychotic) drugs, was first described in 1957 (1, 2). During the past fifteen years this syndrome has come to the medicolegal forefront since numerous lawsuits have appeared on behalf of patients who developed TD as a consequence of neuroleptic therapy. In addition, TD has posed a major clinical and ethical dilemma for practicing physicians who wish to provide quality medical care to patients with chronic psychiatric disorders while also mitigating the risk of untreatable side effects. Concerns about TD arise largely because of its rather high prevalence, estimated at approximately 15 to 20 percent of patients exposed chronically to neuroleptics (3); the fact that it is presently untreatable; and, of greatest concern to most clinicians, the belief that it is frequently irreversible.

TD has been studied extensively in the past 20 years, with early research focusing mostly on epidemiology and attempts to treat the condition, while little attention was paid to the natural course of the illness. Older reports on the clinical course of TD are limited largely by the short duration of follow-up, usually 1 year or less. More recently, some long-term follow-up studies have been reported. While

---

This work was conducted by the author while a member of the full-time faculty at the State University of New York at Syracuse and a staff physician at the Syracuse Veterans Administration Medical Center, and prior to his association with Ciba-Geigy Corporation. As such, it reflects the author's privately held opinions while he worked at the State University of New York and the Veterans Administration and does not represent the opinions of Ciba-Geigy Corporation.

patient populations and methodologies have differed, these studies can help to characterize the course and outcome for patients who develop TD during neuroleptic therapy.

In addition some of these studies include reports on patients who were withdrawn from neuroleptic therapy as well as those who continued neuroleptic therapy. These studies are important, since it has been widely believed that reversibility of TD is related to discontinuation of neuroleptics; that is, TD may be reversible if neuroleptics are discontinued but it will inevitably become irreversible, or even progressive, if neuroleptics are continued. This belief has led to the recommendation that all patients with TD be given a trial off neuroleptic drugs. Although this advice is rational because it encourages discontinuation of drug treatment when this is no longer necessary to control psychotic symptoms, it has created a dilemma for many physicians treating patients for whom neuroleptic discontinuation leads to a relapse of the underlying psychotic disorder. For such patients the risk of psychotic relapse may outweigh the risk of permanent or progressive TD, thus justifying continued neuroleptic therapy for the psychotic disorder. On the other hand, while the milder forms of TD are disfiguring at most, the more severe forms of TD can be very disabling (4, 5). Faced with this dilemma, the physician and patient will benefit greatly from a treatment strategy based on empirically determined facts about the long-term clinical course of TD.

REVIEW OF FOLLOW-UP STUDIES

A review of all published follow-up studies, including patients who discontinued neuroleptics as well as patients continuing neuroleptics, reveals a range of outcomes. In a few studies TD was unchanged during follow-up, and occasional patients were reported to experience worsening of TD during follow-up. The majority of reports, however, are more favorable, finding that TD may improve, and even remit, over the long term. Thus, the specter of TD necessarily becoming irreversible or gradually progressive is not generally supported by these published reports.

Studies that report long-term clinical observations of patients who discontinued neuroleptic drugs are important because they directly address the issue of benefit, vis-à-vis TD, of drug discontinuation. Although some patients were observed to experience worsening of TD after drug discontinuation, this was often transient, and the majority experienced gradual improvement or at least did not become worse during long-term follow-up. Only a minority of patients had worsening of TD that persisted long after drug discontinuation

(6–12). The studies are reassuring insofar as they support the advised practice of discontinuing neuroleptic drugs, where feasible, for patients who develop TD and permit a reasonably optimistic forecast for these patients over the long term.

A fairly large proportion (estimated to be more than 50 percent) of chronically psychotic patients, however, cannot be maintained off neuroleptic drugs for very long without a significant risk of relapse. Therefore, long-term observation of patients with TD who required continued neuroleptic treatment may be even more valuable in assessing long-term risks and devising useful therapeutic strategies. While such studies have been less frequently reported, they also show a tendency toward improvement or stabilization of TD during long-term follow-up for the majority of patients. Only a few patients experienced worsening of TD while continuing neuroleptic therapy, and a surprisingly large number appeared to have gradually improved over many months or years (8, 10, 13–16).

Thus, worsening of TD appears to be the exception rather than the rule, and in some patients the syndrome appears to be reversible, even on continued neuroleptic therapy. Indeed, if gradual improvement is interpreted as a sign of "reversibility," albeit partial, then one might even conclude that the clinical course of TD during continued neuroleptic treatment is more likely to be persistent, with potential for improvement rather than irreversible.

Because some patients requiring chronic maintenance neuroleptic drug therapy can be expected to remain on medication for many years, it is important to evaluate not only the short-term course (1 year or less) but also the long-term course (several years) of TD. For those studies that included follow-up beyond 1 year, further improvements in TD were sometimes observed during subsequent years among patients continuing neuroleptic at the same or reduced dose as well as among patients who discontinued neuroleptic therapy (8, 10, 12, 14). Thus, although the most common course of TD includes short-term improvement, these studies suggest that patients may still show improvement over the long term.

One further comment on these studies seems necessary. The drug discontinuation studies clearly track the natural course of the disease without the confounding variable of concomitant drug treatment that may alter the clinical picture. It is well known that neuroleptic drugs, themselves causative for TD, nevertheless are capable of suppressing the symptoms of TD. Thus, the long-term follow-up studies of patients continuing neuroleptics may be reporting on symptoms of TD that are partially suppressed or "masked" by the continued neuroleptic treatment. It could be argued, therefore, that these studies do not accurately estimate the true severity of the patient's movement disorder. Notwithstanding this methodologic problem, the accumulated evidence still indicates that TD does not inevitably worsen when neuroleptic drugs are continued and provides a rational basis for continuing neuroleptic treatment in patients who cannot tolerate drug withdrawal.

INTRODUCTION TO THE PRESENT STUDY

This report is of clinical observations only. Although the study was undertaken with certain a priori hypotheses and was conducted in a rigorous fashion with respect to consistency of clinical ratings and the use of a carefully designed clinical protocol, it lacks the scientific rigor of controlled clinical studies. This limitation may also be a virtue, however, since the data reflect observations emanating from clinical practice and therefore may more closely approximate the actual conditions and circumstances faced by other clinicians in their practices.

In 1978 I started a Tardive Dyskinesia Clinic at the Syracuse Veterans Administration Medical Center. Patients with various movement disorders were evaluated on referral from the hospital's inpatient services and outpatient clinics. In addition, I provided the identical consultation to nonveterans within the State University of New York Upstate Medical Center in Syracuse. During the period 1978 to 1985 more than 300 patients were seen in consultation. With few exceptions, these patients had neuroleptic-induced tardive dyskinesia. A large majority of these patients received follow-up from the referring physician or clinic with only occasional reevaluation in the Tardive Dyskinesia Clinic. The remainder received regular follow-up in the clinic for varying periods of time. This chapter includes data obtained from 42 patients who had tardive dyskinesia and were followed regularly in the clinic for at least 1 year. Patients with other movement disorders are not included. In addition, patients who were taking medications other than neuroleptics, or had other potentially complicating medical illnesses, have been excluded from this report.

The study was undertaken with two basic hypotheses: 1) that patients maintained chronically on neuroleptic drugs could be maintained on substantially reduced doses without significant risk of relapse, and 2) that TD on a long-term basis would improve with reduction or discontinuation of neuroleptic drug and worsen with continuation or increase of neuroleptic drug.

METHOD

The diagnosis of tardive dyskinesia was made using the following criteria: 1) a history of neuroleptic drug exposure of at least 4 weeks; 2) presence of abnormal involuntary movements characteristic of TD, determined by clinical examination; 3) abnormal movements not due to other drug therapies; 4) abnormal movements not due to other neurologic disease (for example, Huntington's disease, Wilson's disease, Gilles de la Tourette's syndrome); and 5) abnormal movements not due to other systemic disease (for example, hyperthyroidism).

Patients receiving antiparkinson drugs were withdrawn from these drugs for 1 week before baseline evaluation. Patients with concomitant TD and parkinsonism were excluded from this study. All evaluations were conducted by the author.

Baseline evaluation (at initial visit or 1 week after withdrawal of antiparkinson drugs) included a mental status examination, a complete physical and neurological examination, the Abnormal Involuntary Movement Scale (AIMS) (17), and laboratory studies (necessary to rule out other causes of movement disorder).

Follow-up evaluations were conducted at weekly intervals for 12 weeks and at least quarterly thereafter, depending on the clinical state of the patient. These evaluations included a mental status examination, the AIMS, and Clinical Global Impression of change on a 7-point scale (much improved, moderately improved, minimally improved, no change, minimally worse, moderately worse, much worse).

Neuroleptic withdrawal was accomplished on the following schedule: If mental status permitted, the neuroleptic dose was immediately reduced by 25 to 33 percent. Further reductions of dose by 25 to 33 percent were accomplished at weekly intervals if mental status permitted. Where mental status changes precluded weekly dose reductions, the previous dose was maintained and further dose reductions were subsequently attempted as tolerated by the patient. If the clinical condition warranted, dose escalations could also be introduced as needed. It must be emphasized that rigid adherence to the dose reduction schedule was not the primary aim of the study and that the patient's clinical conditions determined both the amount and frequency of dose reductions. Nevertheless, many patients were able to follow this schedule and significantly reduce or discontinue the neuroleptic drug rather rapidly. None of the patients required escalation of drug dose during the period of study.

The duration of follow-up was not predetermined and depended entirely on clinical need. Thus, patients were followed for varying periods of time, ranging from 1 to more than 5 years.

PATIENT CHARACTERISTICS

Forty-two patients entered the study and were followed for at least 1 year. They included 39 men and 3 women (the disproportionately large number of male patients was because of the majority of patients being referred through the Veterans Administration Medical Center). Although most carried a diagnosis of schizophrenia, several other diagnoses were represented in this sample (paranoia, one; organic brain syndrome, five; bipolar disorder, one; depression, three; and gastrointestinal disorder with no psychiatric diagnosis, one). Mean age at entry was 52 years (SD = 11.6, range = 22–73) and mean AIMS score at baseline was 18.6 (SD = 7.8, range = 7–41). Nineteen of the original 42 patients were seen at 2-year follow-up, 15 at 3-year follow-up, 9 at 4-year follow-up, and 6 of the original 42 patients were followed for 5 years or more.

No effort was made to assign the patients to a particular treatment strategy. Instead, an attempt was made to withdraw all patients from neuroleptic drug as tolerated based on clinical condition. Subgroups were determined a posteriori, based on both treatment and outcome variables. Three subgroups were identified from treatment variables: neuroleptic drug discontinued, neuroleptic dose reduced, and neuroleptic dose unchanged (no patients required increased doses). Four subgroups were identified from outcome variables: TD remitted, TD improved, TD unchanged, and TD worsened. The characteristics and distribution of patients in each subgroup are shown in Tables 1 and 2. For purposes of definition, the group identified as neuroleptic dose reduced were required to achieve at least a 25 percent reduction of dose from baseline. In fact, the majority of patients in this group could be maintained on 50 percent or less of their baseline neuroleptic dose. The outcome variable groups were determined by the Clinical Global Impression; that is, any degree of improvement or worsening on this scale was sufficient for inclusion in the corresponding outcome group. The global impressions corresponded to a minimum change of 3 points on the AIMS; thus, a clinical impression of minimally improved was always accompanied by a reduction of 3 or more points on the AIMS and minimally worse was accompanied by at least a 3-point increase in the AIMS score. The classification by subgroup was made based on ratings at the last follow-up visit. Although some patients showed fluctuations in their clinical course that will not be revealed by this method of classification, overall the changes were not substantial from visit to visit except in the period immediately following a reduction in dose, at which time there often was a brief worsening which was usually followed by improvement. Almost universally, the involuntary movements tended to stabilize after a period of time and intervisit AIMS ratings for an individual patient were remarkably similar during the later follow-up visits.

As can be seen from Table 1, 25 patients (60 percent) tolerated discontinuation of neuroleptic drug without psychotic relapse. An additional eight patients could achieve a substantial reduction of neuroleptic dose and only nine patients could not tolerate dose reduction. These subgroups did not differ significantly by age, although the older patients seemed to be more tolerant of dose reduction or discontinuation of drug. There were no differences among these three groups in baseline AIMS scores.

From Table 2 it can be seen that six patients had complete remission of TD. Approximately half of the patients either remitted or improved in TD symptoms, while half were unchanged or worsened. It is also worth emphasizing that only 3 of these 42 patients showed worsening of TD. Patients experiencing remission and improvement of TD tended to be younger than patients with no improvement or worsening of TD. Mean baseline AIMS scores were not significantly

Table 1. Treatment variable subgroups.

Neuroleptic	n	%	Mean age ± SD	Mean AIMS[a] score at baseline ± D
Discontinued	25	60	54.2 ± 9.7	19.0 ± 8.5
Dose reduced	8	19	51.8 ± 13.7	18.1 ± 7.6
Dose unchanged	9	21	46.3 ± 13.2	18.1 ± 6.6

[a]Abnormal Involuntary Movement Scale.

Table 2. Outcome variable subgroups.

Tardive dyskinesia	n	%	Mean age ± SD	Mean AIMS[a] score at baseline ± SD
Remitted	6	14	48.2 ± 12.0	16.0 ± 3.1
Improved	14	33	51.1 ± 9.5	17.9 ± 8.8
Unchanged	19	45	53.2 ± 13.1	20.7 ± 7.7
Worsened	3	7	56.7 ± 3.7	14.0 ± 6.2

[a]Abnormal Involuntary Movement Scale.

different among these groups, although patients whose TD was un-changed during follow-up had the highest AIMS scores at baseline.

Table 3 provides a matrix comparing the same group of 42 patients on both treatment variables and outcome variables. From Table 3 it can be seen that only patients who discontinued drug showed re-mission of TD; that is, no patients who continued neuroleptic (dose either reduced or unchanged) experienced remission of TD. Al-though more than half of the neuroleptic discontinuation group either improved or remitted, nearly half were unchanged or worse, and two of the three patients in this study whose TD worsened were among the neuroleptic discontinuation group. Similarly, half of the patients with neuroleptic dose reduction improved (although none had remission) and half were unchanged or worse. One patient in the neuroleptic dose reduction group experienced worsening of TD. Among the group with neuroleptic dose unchanged, one-third im-proved and two-thirds were unchanged. None of the patients in this group had worsening of TD.

Figure 1 illustrates changes in TD (mean AIMS scores) during the first year of follow-up for all 42 patients in the three subgroups determined by treatment variables. As can be seen from the figure, all patients showed improvement during the first year, with the patients having drug discontinuation showing the largest and most rapid decline in AIMS scores. Figure 2 similarly illustrates changes

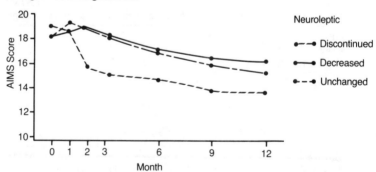

Figure 1. Changes in tardive dyskinesia (TD) (mean scores on the Ab-normal Involuntary Movement Scale (AIMS)) during the first year of follow-up for the three treatment variable subgroups: neuroleptic discontinued, neuroleptic decreased, and neuroleptic unchanged (n = 42).

Table 3. Change in tardive dyskinesia.

Neuroleptic	n	%	Remitted		Improved		Unchanged		Worsened	
			n	%	n	%	n	%	n	%
Discontinued	25	60	6	24	7	28	10	40	2	8
Reduced	8	19	0		4	50	3	38	1	13
Unchanged	9	21	0		3	33	6	67	0	
Total			6	14	14	33	19	45	3	7

Change in TD During First Year

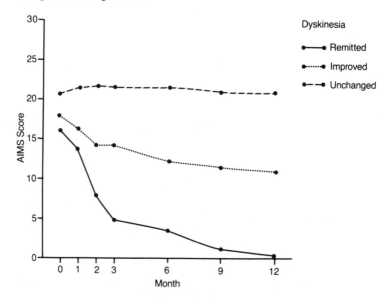

Figure 2. Changes in tardive dyskinesia (TD) (mean scores on the Abnormal Involuntary Movement Scale (AIMS)) during the first year of follow-up for three outcome variable subgroups: TD remitted, TD improved, and TD unchanged (n = 39). Three patients whose TD worsened are not included.

in AIMS scores during the first year of follow-up for the 39 patients in the outcome variable subgroups: remitted, improved, or unchanged (the three patients for whom AIMS scores increased are not represented on Figure 2). As Figure 2 illustrates, those patients experiencing improvement, but not remission, of TD tended to improve gradually over the course of 1 year, while the patients experiencing remission of TD did so fairly rapidly, with the majority of improvement occurring within 6 to 9 months, and remission in all patients occurring within 12 months.

Figure 3 illustrates the course of clinical improvement during the first year for each of the six patients experiencing remission of TD. Here it can be seen that five of the six patients were essentially symptom free by 6 months and only one of the patients had significant symptoms persisting beyond 6 months after withdrawal of neuroleptic drug.

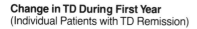

Change in TD During First Year
(Individual Patients with TD Remission)

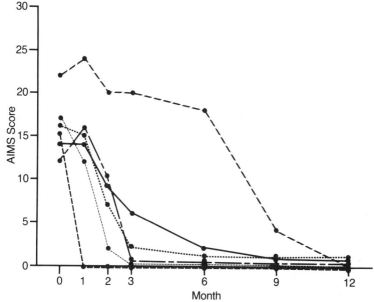

Figure 3.   Changes in tardive dyskinesia (TD) (scores on the Abnormal Involuntary Movement Scale (AIMS)) for six patients showing remission of TD during the first year of treatment.

Scores on the AIMS for those patients who were followed for 2, 3, 4, and 5 years are shown in Figures 4 and 5. Figure 4 shows the changes in mean AIMS scores for only those patients whose TD improved during the first and subsequent years. Patients with TD remission are not included in Figure 4 since all remissions occurred during the first 12 months; that is, no additional patients experienced complete remission for the first time during years 2 through 5 of follow-up. Those patients whose TD remitted during the first year and who were followed subsequently also did not have any reemergence of TD symptoms. As Figure 4 shows, patients with improvement in TD continued to improve during the second year of follow-up but further improvement was not observed during the third, fourth, and fifth year of follow-up. Since patients who left the study before 3-, 4-, and 5-year follow-up were not evaluated at these time points, it is unknown whether further changes in TD occurred subsequently. What these data show is that those patients followed for

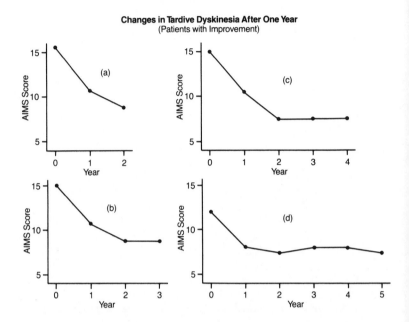

Figure 4. Changes in tardive dyskinesia (mean scores on the Abnormal Involuntary Movement Scale (AIMS)) during long-term follow-up for patients showing improvement (excluding patients with remission): (a) patients followed for 2 years (n = 7), (b) patients followed for 3 years (n = 7), (c) patients followed for 4 years (n = 4), and (d) patients followed for 5 years (n = 2).

more than 2 years showed maximal improvement at 2 years and then stabilized for the remainder of the follow-up period of evaluation. Figure 5 illustrates the changes in AIMS scores for those patients followed longer than 1 year and compares patients continuing on neuroleptic drug with those who discontinued neuroleptic drug. It is evident from Figure 5 that patients discontinuing neuroleptic did not have further improvement in TD symptoms after the first year of follow-up, and that the continued improvement in TD observed between year 1 and year 2 occurred primarily in those patients who continued to receive neuroleptic drugs, either at the same or reduced dose. Furthermore, no additional improvement in TD was observed after 2 years in either group (neuroleptic continued or discontinued). In addition, since several of the patients with TD remission were not followed for 2 years or more, they are not included in Figure 5.

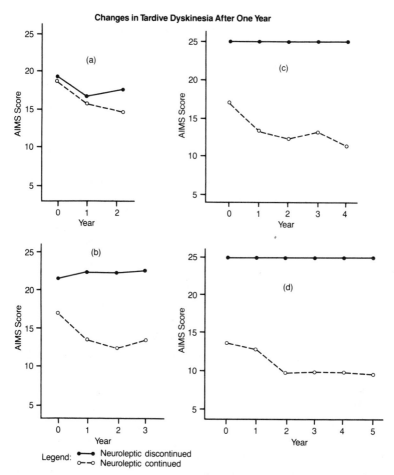

Figure 5. Changes in tardive dyskinesia (mean scores on the Abnormal Involuntary Movement Scale (AIMS)) during long-term follow-up for patients continuing or discontinuing neuroleptic drug: (a) patients followed for 2 years (continued n = 7, discontinued n = 12), (b) patients followed for 3 years (continued n = 6, discontinued n = 9), (c) patients followed for 4 years (continued n = 6, discontinued n = 3), (d) patients followed for 5 years (continued n = 3, discontinued n = 3).

Thus, it can be seen that the substantial improvement in the drug discontinuation group during the first year (Figure 1) is largely attributable to patients whose TD remitted.

DISCUSSION

This long-term follow-up study of 42 patients with tardive dyskinesia found that more than half (60 percent) of the patients could be withdrawn from neuroleptic drug and maintained for a prolonged period of follow-up (1 to 5 years) without adverse consequences. An additional 19 percent could be maintained at substantially reduced doses (usually less than half of what had been prescribed at the time of study entry), while 21 percent required maintenance at the originally prescribed dose. Among those who discontinued neuroleptic, six patients had complete remission of TD within 1 year, while no patients continuing neuroleptics experienced remission. Improvements in TD during the first year of follow-up were of greater magnitude and occurred more rapidly among patients who discontinued neuroleptic, while more gradual improvement also occurred during the first year among patients who continued to receive neuroleptic drugs, whether the dose was reduced or unchanged. Among patients followed more than 1 year, further improvement was seen primarily among those who continued neuroleptic, whereas those who had been withdrawn from neuroleptic appeared to show maximal improvement at 1 year and no further improvement at subsequent follow-up evaluations. In this study, approximately half of patients showed remission or improvement of TD during long-term follow-up, and these patients tended to be younger than the patients whose TD was unchanged or worse. A more favorable prognosis for improvement in TD among younger patients has been found in several other studies (11, 12, 18–21). There were only three patients whose TD became worse: one patient who continued neuroleptic at a reduced dose and two patients whose neuroleptic drug was withdrawn. None of the patients who continued neuroleptic with dose unchanged experienced worsening of TD.

Because the study was designed to make drug dose adjustments based on the clinical condition of the patient, it is not possible to assess from this study what the risk of relapse might be in any patient population withdrawn from neuroleptic drugs; however, an attempt was made to withdraw neuroleptics from all patients in this study. Only 17 (40 percent) of these patients required continued neuroleptic treatment and only 9 patients (21 percent) required that the original dose be maintained during the course of this study. Of course, it is possible that with longer follow-up, additional need for neuroleptic might have been discovered among those patients who were discontinued or had dose reductions. In addition, it should be emphasized that this study included a specific population that was mostly male, mostly drawn from a Veterans Administration health care setting, and referred for evaluation of movement disorder. Results from this group may not be generalizable to other patient populations.

CONCLUSIONS

The results of this study indicate that neuroleptic drug discontinuation or dose reduction may be well tolerated by a substantial proportion of patients (more than half) who have been chronically treated with these drugs. Although all of these patients had TD when entering the study, this finding suggests that many patients are receiving neuroleptic medication that no longer provides real benefit. If this is also true for patients without TD then it suggests that many patients could have the risk of TD reduced by a careful evaluation of their continuing need for a neuroleptic drug. For those patients who already have developed TD, the results of this study suggest that remission of TD is more likely with discontinuation of neuroleptics; in fact, no patient maintained on neuroleptic in this study experienced TD remission. Furthermore, improvement of TD during the first year was of greatest magnitude and occurred most rapidly among those who discontinued neuroleptic. On the other hand, patients who continued neuroleptics (at the same or reduced dose) also showed improvement in TD symptoms during long-term follow-up. Thus, it appears that TD does not worsen and in fact may continue to improve even with continued neuroleptic drug treatment. While the recommendation to attempt dose reduction and/or withdrawal of neuroleptic in patients with TD remains appropriate and may benefit a majority of patients, it also appears that continuing neuroleptic drugs, where indicated to control psychosis, does not lead to an inevitable worsening of TD; nor does it prevent the eventual improvement of TD symptoms. Clinicians faced with the dilemma of chronic psychosis in a patient with TD could feel comfortable continuing to treat the psychosis with neuroleptic drugs without fear of aggravating the TD in the majority of patients. Of course, it will remain paramount in such cases that the continuing need for neuroleptic drug be proved, establishing a favorable risk–benefit ratio, in order to fully justify this treatment strategy.

Finally, although this study was designed to continue neuroleptic treatment only where needed to control psychosis and thus did not evaluate the relationship between persistence of TD and persistence of psychosis, the study does suggest that patients who continue to require neuroleptics are at higher risk for persistence of TD than patients who can discontinue neuroleptics. Whether the increased persistence of TD in these patients is related solely to neuroleptic treatment or is related to the persistence of the underlying psychosis, or possibly to an interaction of the two, is an important research question that deserves further study.

REFERENCES

1. Schonecker M: Beitrag zu der Mitteilung von Kulenkampff und Tarnow. Ein eighentumliches syndrom im oralen bereich bei megaphenapplikation. Nervenarzt 28–35, 1957 (for English translation see reference 2)

2. DeVeaugh-Geiss J (ed): Tardive Dyskinesia and Related Involuntary Movement Disorders. Boston, Wright-PSG, 1982, pp. 199–201 (English translation of Schonecker 1957)

3. American Psychiatric Association: Tardive Dyskinesia: Task Force Report 18. Washington, DC, American Psychiatric Association, 1980

4. Casey DE: Tardive dyskinesia as a life-threatening illness. Am J Psychiatry 135:486–488, 1978

5. Wolf ME, Mosnaim AD: Identifying subtypes of tardive dyskinesia. Hosp Community Psychiatry 35:828–830, 1984

6. Branchey MH, Branchey LB, Richardson MA: Effects of neuroleptic adjustment on clinical condition and tardive dyskinesia in schizophrenic patients. Am J Psychiatry 138:608–612, 1981

7. Carpenter WT, Rey AC, Stephens JH: Covert dyskinesia in ambulatory schizophrenia. Lancet 2:212–213, 1980

8. Casey DE, Povlsen UJ, Meidahl B, et al: Neuroleptic-induced tardive dyskinesia and parkinsonism: changes during several years of continuing treatment. Psychopharmacol Bull 22:250–253, 1986

9. Crane GE: Persistence of neurological symptoms due to neuroleptic drugs. Am J Psychiatry 127:1407–1410, 1971

10. Gardos G, Cole JO, Perenyi A, et al: Five-year follow-up study of tardive dyskinesia, in Chronic Treatments in Neuropsychiatry. Edited by Kemali D, Racagni G. New York, Raven, 1985, pp. 37–42

11. Jeste DV, Potkin SG, Sinha S, et al: Tardive dyskinesia—reversible and persistent. Arch Gen Psychiatry 36:585–590, 1979

12. Yassa R, Nair V, Schwartz G: Tardive dyskinesia: a two-year follow-up study. Psychosomatics 25:852–855, 1984

13. Barron ET, McCreadie RG: One year follow-up of tardive dyskinesia. Br J Psychiatry 143:423–424, 1983

14. Chouinard G, Annable L, Mercier P, et al: A five-year follow-up study of tardive dyskinesia. Psychopharmacol Bull 22:259–263, 1986

15. Kalachnik JE, Harder SR, Kidd-Nielsen P, et al: Persistent tardive dyskinesia in randomly assigned neuroleptic reduction, neuroleptic non-reduction and no-neuroleptic history groups: preliminary results. Psychopharmacol Bull 20:27–32, 1984

16. Kane JM, Woerner M, Sarantakos S, et al: Do low dose neuroleptics prevent or ameliorate tardive dyskinesia? in Tardive Dyskinesia and Neuroleptics: From Dogma to Reason. Edited by Casey DE, Gardos G. Washington, DC, American Psychiatric Press, 1986, pp. 99–107

17. Guy W (ed): ECDEU Assessment Manual for Psychopharmacology (U.S. Department of Health, Education and Welfare Publication No. 76-338). Washington, DC, U.S. Government Printing Office, 1976

18. Seeman MV: Tardive dyskinesia: two-year recovery. Compr Psychiatry 22:189–192, 1981

19. Smith JM, Baldessarini RJ: Changes in prevalence, severity and recovery in tardive dyskinesia with age. Arch Gen Psychiatry 37:1368–1373, 1980

20. Smith JM, Burke MP, Moon CO: Long-term changes in AIMS ratings and their relation to medication history. Psychopharmacol Bull 17:120–121, 1981

21. Yagi G, Itoh H: A 10-year follow-up study of tardive dyskinesia—with special reference to the influence of neuroleptic administration on the long-term prognosis. Keio J Med 34:211–219, 1985

Chapter 8

Contrasts Between Patients' Characteristics Associated with Tardive Dyskinesia versus Those Associated with Parkinsonism-Like Symptoms

Mary Ann Richardson, Ph.D.
Raymond Pass, Ph.D.
Zachary Bregman, M.D.

Chapter 8

Contrasts Between Patients' Characteristics Associated with Tardive Dyskinesia versus Those Associated with Parkinsonism-Like Symptoms

P sychiatric patients treated with neuroleptics can manifest a range of neurological syndromes considered to be secondary to this treatment, the most common of these being tardive dyskinesia (TD) and parkinsonism-like symptoms (PK). These two disorders can be seen singly in patients or be found to coexist (1, 2). Younger male patients are more likely to show the disorders singly, while older female patients are more likely to exhibit coexisting TD and PK (3). The present study was conducted among young male schizophrenic patients in an effort to define patient characteristics associated with the presence of TD and PK in a single body of patients. The investigation was stimulated by prior work in three general areas: 1) the associations reported between TD and affective symptoms both positive (2, 4–8) and negative (9, 10), 2) the associations reported between Parkinson's disease and depression (11–13), and 3) the controversy over whether the depression seen in schizophrenia is part of the disease process or a neuroleptic side effect (14–16).

METHOD

Subjects

During a 4-month period at a state psychiatric center, chart-diagnosed male schizophrenic patients (ages 18 to 44) with no less than 3 years and no more than 20 years since their first neuroleptic treatment were screened for possible study inclusion. Patients were excluded from the study if they were not English speaking, were mute or deaf, were incompetent to give consent or refused consent, failed to satisfy criteria from the *Diagnostic and Statistical Manual of Mental Disorders (Third Edition;* [17] *DSM-III)* or Research Diagnostic Criteria for schizophrenia at a lifetime diagnostic interview, or did not have a hospital stay long enough to complete study procedures.

Procedure

Prior to the diagnostic interview, patient charts were reviewed to collect a lifetime symptom profile. During the interview, data were collected on significant factors from the patient history. After fulfilling diagnostic criteria, the patients were evaluated by the first author for TD by use of the Simpson Abbreviated Dyskinesia Scale (ADS) (18) and placed into either a case group (n = 16) (positive for TD) or a control group (n = 16) (negative for TD). The positive TD designation was given to those patients surpassing a criterion measure indicating at least mild TD. The measure was a global rating based on the following ADS items: lip movements, chewing movements, lateral jaw movements, bon-bon sign, tongue protrusion, choreo/athetoid tongue movements, axial hyperkinesia, and choreo/athetoid finger, wrist, ankle, or toe movements. Evaluations for parkinsonism-like symptoms were performed (also by the first author) by use of the Simpson-Angus Neurological Rating Scale (19). Based on a criterion measure of an average score of 0.4 on all 10 scale items, patients were placed in a case group (n = 7) (positive for PK) or a control group (n = 25) (negative for PK). Two raters (second and third authors), blind to the TD or PK side effect status, interviewed the patients at different points in time and assessed them using the Hamilton Psychiatric Rating Scale for Depression (HAM-D) (20), the Brief Psychiatric Rating Scale (BPRS) (21), and the Affective Flattening Scale (AFS) (22). The study measure used for each scale was the average of the two ratings. One of the raters also administered the Mini-Mental State Exam (MMSE) (23), and a single score was used for that scale. For 20 of the patients, a telephone interview of a family member was conducted to collect information regarding any family history of psychiatric illness. The Family History Research Diagnostic Criteria (24) was used for this assessment.

Statistical Analyses

The variables collected from the diagnostic interview were tested for significant association with TD or PK by use of the chi-square statistic. Univariate associations between side effect status on the one hand, and demographic and psychometric variables on the other, were tested for significance with either a t test or a Mann-Whitney U test, whichever was appropriate. An odds ratio was calculated for the family history information to demonstrate the degree of association between the antecedent event of a positive family history and the outcome event of TD or PK. The ratio is an estimate of the relative risk of developing TD when a family history of psychiatric illness is present. Confidence intervals and a Fischer-Owen exact test were employed for significance testing of this odds ratio (25).

RESULTS

Demographic Variables

The demographic study variables—age, time since first neuroleptic treatment, chlorpromazine (CPZ) equivalent dose at evaluation, and length of current admission—showed differing patterns for TD and PK (see Figures 1 through 4). TD was positively associated with the

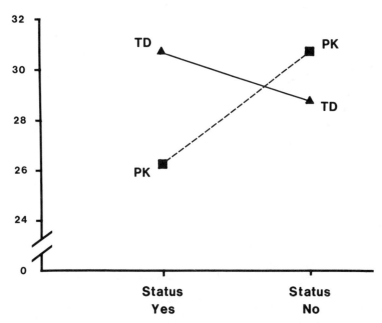

Figure 1. Mean age of subjects. t tests: TD yes vs. TD no, t = 0.83, ns; PK yes vs. PK no, t = 1.98, ns.

length of the current admission while PK showed a significant negative association with that variable. TD status also showed a significant positive relationship to the time since first neuroleptic treatment while PK was not significantly associated with this treatment variable.

Clinical Status Evaluations

Figure 5 and Table 1 demonstrate the marked contrasts between TD and PK status for the BPRS. The total BPRS score (Figure 5) showed a significant positive association with TD status while no association with total score was seen for PK. Further, an item analysis (Table 1) demonstrated that there was no overlap between items associated with TD status (seven items) and those associated with PK status (two items).

Results on the HAM-D total score (Figure 6 and Table 2) contrasted with those for the BPRS total score. There was no association between the HAM-D total score (Figure 6) and TD, but there was a significant positive association between this score and PK. As with the BPRS, there was no overlap between the significant HAM-D

YEARS

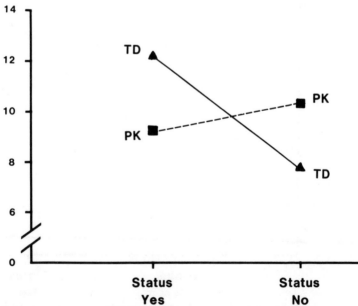

Figure 2. Time since first neuroleptic treatment. t tests: TD yes vs. TD no, t = 3.45, p ≤ .01; PK yes vs. PK no, t = 0.64, ns.

items associated with PK (six items) and those associated with TD (two items) (Table 2).

Neither the total AFS score (TD yes versus TD no, U = 109.0, ns; PK yes versus PK no, U = 95.0, ns nor the MMSE score (TD yes versus TD no, t = 0.6, ns; PK yes versus PK no, t = 0.6, ns) were significantly associated with either side effect. The Inappropriate Affect item of the AFS was, however, positively associated with TD (TD yes versus TD no, U = 54.0, p ≤ .01).

Psychiatric History Data

The study variables that were derived from the chart review and diagnostic interview also demonstrated marked contrasts between TD status and PK status associations. Figure 7 demonstrates the significant positive relationship for TD with a history of manic symptoms with no association for PK status. Neither TD nor PK were associated with a history of depressive symptoms (TD yes versus TD no, X^2 = 0.26, ns; PK yes versus PK no, X^2 = 0.84, ns).

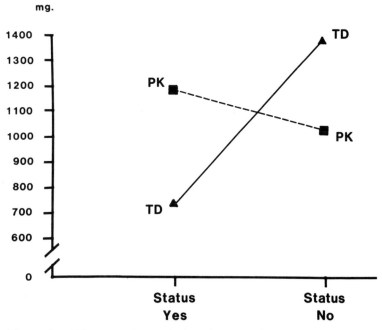

Figure 3. Chlorpromazine equivalent dose at evaluation. t tests: TD yes vs. TD no, t = 1.72, ns; PK yes vs PK no, t = 0.40, ns.

Figure 8 shows opposing significant associations for TD and PK for *DSM-III* defined delusions other than those classified as persecutory or jealous (positive for TD, negative for PK). Neither TD nor PK was associated with a history of persecutory or jealous delusions (TD yes versus TD no, X^2 = 0.16, ns; PK yes versus PK no, X^2 = 0.96, ns).

The odds ratios based on the family psychiatric history data (Figure 9) were not significant when tested using confidence interval methods or a Fischer exact test. The families of those with PK do present a different descriptive profile, however, than the families of those with TD. The strongest relationship shown for TD was with major affective disorder (odds ratio = 4.00) while that for a family history of schizophrenia demonstrated a ratio of 1.0, indicating no relationship. In contrast, for PK the strongest relationship was with a family history of minor psychiatric illness (odds ratio = 0.11) while that for a family history of schizophrenia demonstrated a ratio of 2.22.

YEARS

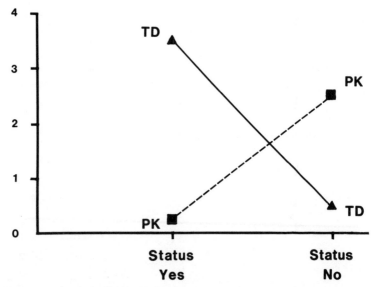

Figure 4.   Length of current admission. t tests: TD yes vs. TD no, t = 2.60, $p \le .05$; PK yes vs. PK no, t = 2.85, $p \le .01$.

Summary

Table 3 shows a summary of the significant associations for all three sets of variables—demographic, clinical status, and psychiatric history—with TD and PK.

DISCUSSION

The data generated from the clinical status evaluations demonstrated marked contrasts between the psychiatric symptom associations for TD status versus those for PK status. A positive TD status showed a strong relationship with psychopathology as assessed by the BPRS whereas a positive PK status was primarily associated with depression as measured by the HAM-D. Although TD status was not significantly related to the total HAM-D, an affective pattern of associations with the disorder can be inferred from the BPRS item analysis in a psychomotor acceleration/manic direction. A positive TD status also was significantly related to the Inappropriate Affect item of the AFS. The lack of association for PK with the AFS casts doubt that a PK-

MEAN TOTAL SCORE

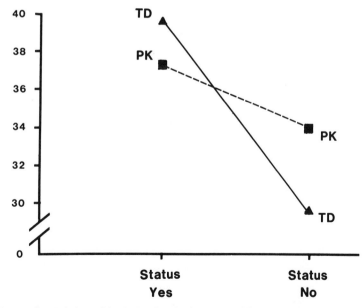

Figure 5. Brief Psychiatric Rating Scale. Mann-Whitney U tests: TD yes vs. TD no, U = 94.0, p ≤ .01; PK yes vs. PK no, U = 64.0, ns.

Table 1. Mean item scores on the Brief Psychiatric Rating Scale and significant associations with side effect status.

Items	TD yes vs. TD no			PK yes vs. PK no		
	Yes	No	$p \leqslant^a$	Yes	No	$p \leqslant^a$
1. Somatic Concern	2.2	1.6	.05			
2. Anxiety				3.1	1.8	.01
4. Conceptual Disorganization	3.6	1.9	.01			
6. Tension	2.9	2.0	.05			
7. Mannerisms/Posturing	1.4	1.0	.01			
10. Hostility	1.8	1.2	.05			
12. Hallucinatory Behavior				3.9	2.3	.05
15. Unusual Thought Content	3.1	1.9	.01			
17. Excitement	2.1	1.3	.01			

Note. TD = tardive dyskinesia, PK = parkinsonism-like symptoms.
[a]Mann-Whitney U test.

MEAN TOTAL SCORE

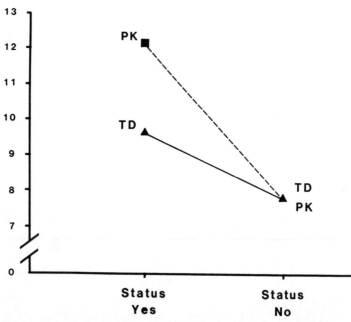

Figure 6. Hamilton Psychiatric Rating Scale for Depression. Mann-Whitney U tests: TD yes vs. TD no, U = 89.5, ns; PK yes vs. PK no, U = 43.5, $p \leqslant .05$.

Table 2. Mean item scores on the Hamilton Psychiatric Rating Scale for Depression and significant associations with side effect status.

Items	TD yes vs. TD no			PK yes vs. PK no		
	Yes	No	$p \leqslant$[a]	Yes	No	$p \leqslant$[a]
2. Guilt				0.9	0.4	.05
4. Suicide	0.9	0.3	.05			
10. Anxiety—Psychic				1.5	0.7	.05
11. Anxiety—Somatic				0.5	0.2	.05
12. Somatic Symptoms—GI				0.9	0.3	.05
14. Genital Symptoms				0.6	0.2	.05
15. Hypochondriasis	0.9	0.3	.01			
17. Insight				0.6	1.3	.01

Note. TD = tardive dyskinesia, PK = parkinsonism-like symptoms.
[a]Mann-Whitney U test.

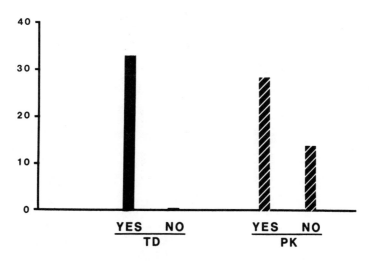

Figure 7. Manic symptoms in history (*Diagnostic and Statistical Manual of Mental Disorders (Third Edition)*). χ^2 tests: TD yes vs. TD no, $\chi^2 = 6.36$, $p \leqslant .05$; PK yes vs. PK no, $\chi^2 = 1.04$, ns.

yes designation in this study was affected by observable akinetic pathology.

The psychiatric history study findings can be interpreted to support the concept of a TD/affective symptom pattern beyond that of a correlational nature, in that 1) there is a demonstrated relationship between TD and manic symptoms as gleaned from the lifetime symptom profile, and 2) there is a fourfold chance of developing TD given a family history of major affective disorders compared to not having such a history. This leads to the conclusion that a vulnerability to develop TD exists in young schizophrenic males who display some affective characteristics.

The psychiatric history data do not, however, support such an extension for PK status in that PK was not associated with a history of major affective disorder. The PK association with depression, therefore, may well represent concurrent neuroleptic side effects as suggested by Galdi (15). An association between HAM-D scores and parkinsonism-like symptoms has been reported previously (26). A caveat is in order, however, in that it has also been reported that

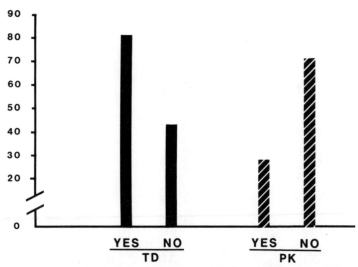

Figure 8. Delusion other than persecutory or jealous (*Diagnostic and Statistical Manual of Mental Disorders (Third Edition)*). χ^2 tests: TD yes vs. TD no, $\chi^2 = 4.80, p \le .05$; PK yes vs. PK no, $\chi^2 = 4.40$, $p \le .05$.

depression in schizophrenia is more likely to be seen early in an admission (16, 27, 28) and PK yes in this study showed a significant negative association with the length of the current admission.

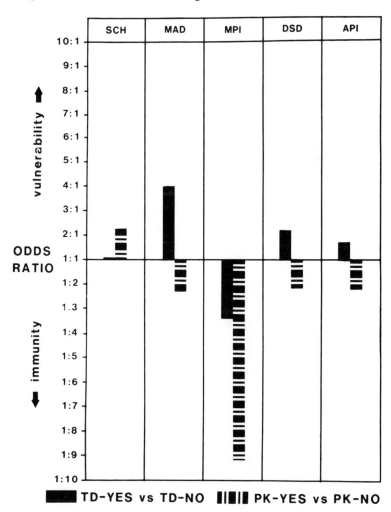

Figure 9.   Family psychiatric history: odds ratio analysis (n = 20). TD = tardive dyskinesia; PK = parkinsonism-like symptoms; SCH = schizophrenia; MAD = major affective disorders; MPI = minor psychiatric illness; DSD = depressive spectrum disorders; API = all psychiatric illness.

Aside from the interpretations as to the meaning and significance of the study findings for PK and TD, it is clear from the study data that these disorders exist within the construct of differing, if not contrasting, patient profiles.

Table 3.   Summary of study associations with side effect status.

Associated with TD Status	Associated with PK Status
Demographic variables	
Years since first treatment	Length of current admission (negative)
Length of current admission	
Clinical status	
Hamilton Scale items	
Suicide	Guilt
Hypochondriasis	Anxiety—Psychic
	Anxiety—Somatic
	Somatic Symptoms—GI
	Genital Symptoms
	Insight (negative)
	Total Scale
Brief Psychiatric Rating Scale items	
Somatic Concern	Anxiety
Conceptual Disorganization	Hallucinatory Behavior
Tension	
Mannerisms and Posturing	
Hostility	
Unusual Thought Content	
Excitement	
Total Scale	
Affective Flattening Scale items	
Inappropriate Affect	
Psychiatric history	
Lifetime Symptom Profile	
Delusions Other than	Delusions Other than Persecutory
Persecutory or Jealous	or Jealous (negative)
DSM-III Defined Manic	
Symptoms	

REFERENCES

1. Richardson MA, Craig TJ: The coexistence of parkinsonism-like symptoms and tardive dyskinesia. Am J Psychiatry 139:341–343, 1982

2. Wolf ME, Chevesich J, Lehrer E, et al: The clinical association of tardive dyskinesia and drug induced parkinsonism. Biol Psychiatry 18: 1181–1188, 1983

3. Richardson MA, Pass ER, Craig TJ, et al: The coexistence of parkinsonism-like symptoms and tardive dyskinesia—revisited, in Biological Psychiatry, 1985. Edited by Shagass C, Josiassen RC, Bridger WH, et al. New York, Elsevier Science Publishing 1986, pp. 1211–1213

4. Davis KL, Berger PA, Hollister LE: Tardive dyskinesia and depressive illness. Psychopharmacol Commun 2:125–130, 1976

5. Cutler NR, Post RM: State-related cyclical dyskinesias in manic depressives. J Clin Psychopharmacol 2:350–354, 1982

6. Rosenbaum AH, Maruta T, Jiang N, et al: Endocrine testing in tardive dyskinesia: preliminary report. Am J Psychiatry 136:102–103, 1979

7. Rush M, Diamond F, Alpert M: Depression as a risk factor in tardive dyskinesia. Biol Psychiatry 17:387–392, 1982

8. Wilson IC, Garbutt JC, Lanier CF, et al: Is there a tardive dysmentia? Schizophr Bull 9:187–192, 1983

9. Glazer W, Moore DC, Brenner LM, et al: Tardive dyskinesia: a discontinuation study. Arch Gen Psychiatry 41:623–627, 1984

10. Itil TM, Reisberg B, Hugue M, et al: Clinical profiles of tardive dyskinesia. Compr Psychiatry 22:282–290, 1981

11. Celesea GG, Wanamaker WM: Psychiatric disturbances in Parkinson's disease. Dis Nerv Syst 33:577–583, 1972

12. Mayeux R, Stern Y, Rosen J, et al: Depression, intellectual impairment and Parkinson's disease. Neurology 31:645–650, 1981

13. Holcomb HH: Parkinsonism and depression: dopaminergic mediation of neuropathologic process in human beings, in The Catecholamines in Psychiatric and Neurologic Disorders. Edited by Lake R, Zeigler M. Boston, Butterworth, 1985

14. Hirsch SR: Depression "revealed" in schizophrenia. Br J Psychiatry 140:421–424, 1982

15. Galdi J: The causality of depression in schizophrenia. Br J Psychiatry 142:621–625, 1983

16. Strain F, Heger R, Kliopera C: The time structure of depressive mood in schizophrenic patients. Acta Psychiatr Scand 65:66–73, 1982

17. American Psychiatric Association: Diagnostic and Statistical Manual of Mental Disorders, Third Edition. Washington, DC, American Psychiatric Association, 1980

18. Simpson GM, Lee JH, Zoubok B, et al: A rating scale for tardive dyskinesia. Psychopharmacol (Berlin) 64:171–179, 1979

19. Simpson GM, Angus JWS: Drug-induced extrapyramidal disorders. Acta Psychiatr Scand (Suppl) 221:1–58, 1970

20. Hamilton M: A rating scale for depression. J Neurol Neurosurg Psychiatry 23:56–62, 1960

21. Overall JE, Gorham DR: The brief psychiatric rating scale. Psychol Rep 10:799–812, 1962

22. Andreasen NC: Affecting flattening and the criteria for schizophrenia. Am J Psychiatry 136:944–947, 1979

23. Folstein MF, Folstein SE, McHugh PR: Mini-mental state, a practical method for grading the cognitive state of patients for the clinician. J Psychiatry Res 12:189–198, 1975

24. Andreasen NC, Endicott J, Spitzer RL, et al: The family history method using diagnostic criteria. Reliability and validity. Arch Gen Psychiatry 34:1229–1235, 1977

25. Fleiss JL: Statistical Methods for Rates and Proportions, second edition. New York, John Wiley & Sons, 1981

26. Johnson DAW: Studies of depressive symptoms in schizophrenia. I. The prevalence of depression and its possible causes. Br J Psychiatry 139:89–101, 1981

27. Knights A, Hirsch SR: "Revealed" depression and drug treatment for schizophrenia. Arch Gen Psychiatry 38:806–811, 1981

28. McGlashan TH, Carpenter WT: An investigation of post-psychotic depression. Am J Psychiatry 133:14–19, 1976

Chapter 9

Tardive Dyskinesia in a Psychogeriatric Population

Ramzy Yassa, M.D.
Christine Nastase, M.D.
Yves Camille, M.D.
Lise Belzile, R.N.

Chapter 9

Tardive Dyskinesia in a Psychogeriatric Population

Since the description of tardive dyskinesia (TD) by Schonecker (1), several studies have been conducted to evaluate predisposing factors to its development. The only consistent factor associated with more severe and persistent TD has been age (2). Other factors, including female sex (3–5), organicity (6–8), drug-free periods (9–11), and affective disorders (7, 12–14), have also been reported to contribute to the development of TD. Recently we confirmed earlier observations that late-onset psychosis patients show significantly higher TD prevalence than early onset psychosis subjects (11, 15–18). Several studies have been conducted comparing the prevalence of TD among neuroleptic-treated and neuroleptic-free psychogeriatric patients (3, 19–29). In the neuroleptic-free geriatric patients, the prevalence of abnormal involuntary movements has been estimated to be about 5 percent (2), compared to 40 percent in neuroleptic-treated geriatric patients (23). The present study was conducted to assess the prevalence of abnormal involuntary movements in a psychogeriatric population admitted for the first time to our unit; these same patients were reassessed 2 years later for the presence or absence of TD.

MATERIALS AND METHODS

The patient population consisted of three groups. Group 1 included new admissions (except for first-time hospitalization) to the psychogeriatric unit at the Douglas Hospital Centre during the 2-year period starting September 1, 1984 (n = 120). To this group were added four patients whose charts were reviewed and who were found not to have received neuroleptic since admission. Thus, the total number in Group 1 was 124. The demographic characteristics of this patient population are presented in Table 1. Group 2 included all the psychogeriatric inpatients (five wards) who were available and consented for an assessment of TD. Al the patients were 65 years or older (n = 146). (For demographic characteristics of this patient population see Table 1.) Group 3 included first-time admissions to the psychogeriatric unit during the period of September 1984 to March 1986 (n = 103).

All the available patients were reexamined during the months of September and October 1986 to assess the presence or absence of TD, blind to their neuroleptic uptake. TD was assessed by the Abnormal Involuntary Movement Scale (AIMS), and the diagnosis of TD was established according to Jeste and Wyatt (4).

RESULTS

Prevalence of Abnormal Involuntary Movements

Of the 124 patients who never received neuroleptics, 5 were found to have abnormal involuntary movements (overall 4 percent; 5.9

Table 1. Demographic Characteristics of the Patient Population

Variables	Group 1 (N = 124)	Group 2 (N = 146)
Mean Age (± SD)		
men	72.7 (±6.8)	73.4 (±4.8)
women	75.6 (±8.5)	76.0 (±4.5)
Primary Diagnosis:		
affective disorder		
men	19	10
women	28	27
paranoid psychosis		
men	6	1
women	10	3
schizophrenia		
men	0	25
women	0	43
senile dementia		
men	19	8
women	25	16
alcoholism		
men	4	2
women	4	9
personality disorder		
men	4	0
women	5	1
mental retardation		
men	0	0
women	0	1

percent of the men and 2.9 percent of the women). The movements were confined to the buccal area and were rated as mild.

In contrast, of the 146 patients treated with neuroleptics, 70 exhibited TD (47.9 percent). The mean age and duration of neuroleptic treatment of the patients without or with TD was 73.3 (SD = ±4.9) and 18.3 years (SD = ±10.1) and 73.5 (SD = ±4.8) and 25.0 years (SD = ±7.7), respectively. The difference in length of neuroleptic treatment was statistically significant (t < 141, df > 4.528, p < 0.001). Thirty-three subjects had mild TD, another 33 had moderate TD, and 4 women had severe TD. All the patients had buccal TD, whereas the limbs were affected in nine patients, and body and limbs in another nine subjects. 58.3 percent of the men had mild TD, compared to 41.3 percent of the women, and the body was affected more in women than in men (32.6 percent versus 12.5 percent, χ^2 = 3.34) but this difference did not reach statistical significance.

Follow-Up of the Newly Admitted Patients

Of the 120 newly admitted patients, 103 had never been admitted for 6 months or more. From the 53 patients who never received neuroleptics, 7 patients were lost to follow-up and 7 died during this period, making the final number of subjects in this group 39. Similarly, 50 patients were found to have received neuroleptics during the study period. From this group, 6 subjects were lost to follow-up and 5 patients died, making the final number in this group 39; the demographic characteistics of the patient population are presented in Table 2. All of the 16 newly admitted patients found to have TD were included in the neuroleptic treated group, showing a TD prevalence of 41 percent. TD affected the buccal area in 15 patients and in addition affected the lower limbs and pelvic area in three and two patients, respectively; one patient had respiratory irregularity and another showed severe foot tapping. TD was rated as mild in 4 patients, moderate in 11, and severe in one subject.

Psychotropic Drug Intake

The details of neuroleptic drug intake are presented in Table 3. Of the various factors compared in Table 3, only the duration of hospitalization was significantly different between TD and non-TD patients (t < 37, df > 3.569, p < 0.001).

Onset of TD as Recorded in the Patients' Files

Of the 16 patients with TD, 12 were found to have a recording of TD in their charts. Of these 12 patients, TD was noted in the first

Table 2. Demographic Characteristics of the Follow-up Patients

Variables	Patients Who Never Received Neuroleptics			Patients Who Received Neuroleptics		
	Men (N = 17)	Women (N = 22)	Total (N = 39)	Men (N = 14)	Women (N = 25)	Total (N = 39)
Age	74.5 ± 6.1	73.9 ± 7.2	74.2 ± 6.6	72.4 ± 6.2	77.7 ± 6.4	75.8 ± 6.8
Duration of follow-up (in months)	20.2 ± 6.1	17.7 ± 5.1	18.8 ± 5.7	17.9 ± 6.4	17.0 ± 6.9	17.3 ± 6.6
Duration in hospital (in months)	13.6 ± 7.4	6.3 ± 3.7	9.5 ± 6.6	13.1 ± 6.6	12.2 ± 8.8	12.5 ± 8.0
Diagnosis						
depression	8	12	20	2	6	8
senile dementia	8	5	13	6	11	17
alcoholism	0	2	2	1	2	3
personality disorder	1	3	4	1	0	1
paranoid psychosis	0	0	0	4	6	10

Table 3. Comparative Study Between TD and Non-TD Patients in Neuroleptic-Treated Subjects (Mean ± SD).

Variables	Non-TD Patients (N = 23)	TD Patients (N = 16)	T test (37 df)
Age	76.8 ± 6.4	74.4 ± 7.2	1
duration of follow-up (in months)	16.6 ± 6.4	20.0 ± 4.8	1
duration of hospitalization (in months)	9.0 ± 6.0	16.9 ± 7.8	3.569 $p<0.001$
total neuroleptic time (in months)	12.7 ± 6.8	14.8 ± 8.3	<1
present dose (in mg CPZ equivalents)	96.7 ± 149.2	110.9 ± 147.5	<1
total neuroleptic intake in gms (CPZ equivalents)	59.3 ± 91.5	74.4 ± 83.9	<1

12 months of treatment in five patients. In seven patients, TD was noted between the 13th and 24th months of the study. Thus, 41.7 percent of patients whose TD was recorded developed it within the first year of neuroleptic therapy.

Neuroleptic Discontinuation

Five subjects developed TD after a mean of 7.4 months of continuous neuroleptic treatment. Neuroleptics were discontinued for a mean of 13.5 months (range = 6 to 22 months). Subjects were assessed monthly with the AIMS; no improvement was noted during the observation period.

DISCUSSION

Our study indicates that abnormal involuntary movements occurred in 4 percent of newly admitted non-neuroleptic-treated psychogeriatric patients, which is in agreement with the estimated 5 percent prevalence reported in a recent literature review (2). When compared to neuroleptic-treated patients (Group 2), the difference in prevalence (4 percent versus 41 percent) was statistically significant. The abnormal involuntary movements were mild and localized in the buccal area. TD, on the other hand, was more severe and affected more body areas.

Patients who were started on neuroleptics during the study period (n = 39, Group 3) had a prevalence of TD almost similar to that of patients who were receiving chronic neuroleptic treatment (41 percent versus 48 percent), in agreement with previous reports indicating that TD is more prevalent when neuroleptics are started late in life (11, 15–18). The findings that TD developed in 39 percent of patients who were started on neuroleptics after age 63 and followed up to 28 months (22) compares well with our 41 percent prevalence of TD after a follow-up period of 24 months. Lieberman et al. (28) found that among 79 subjects with a history of neuroleptic treatment (mean age at first admission, 83; mean duration of neuroleptic exposure, 18 months), 16.5 percent developed TD. Based on a retrospective review of elderly patients, it has been suggested that the incidence of TD among elderly subjects may begin to decline after the first 2 years of neuroleptic exposure (29).

It is of interest that in the control group (those subjects who never received neuroleptics), no patient developed abnormal involuntary movements during the study period, in agreement with the findings reported by other investigators (30, 31). However, Owens et al. describes a similar distribution of abnormal involuntary movements in both treated and nontreated chronic schizophrenic patients (32). Crow et al.(33) have indicated that persistent dyskinesia are more commonly seen in psychotic disorders with poor outcome associated with negative symptoms and cognitive impairment.

Drug factors have been studied extensively to attempt to correlate the present dose, total neuroleptic exposure and duration of neuroleptic treatment, to the presence of TD, without conclusive evidence (4). Our findings that no particular drug factor can be implicated in the development of TD are in agreement with the results of other investigators (4). Aging and female sex have been implicated as factors for the development of TD (2) and abnormal involuntary movements (26). However, in our study these two factors were noncontributory to the development of this side effect.

Organic factors are difficult to assess in a population of geriatric age. We did not measure the subtle elements in each of our patients, but confined ourselves to gross psychopathology. Of the 16 TD patients, 9 had a primary organic diagnosis as compared to 23 who did not (56.3 percent versus 47.8 percent). Thus gross organic psychopathology did not appear to be a factor in the development of TD in our patient population.

Neuroleptic discontinuation was attempted in five patients who developed TD. After a follow up of 13.5 months, none of the patients had a reversal of their TD, in agreement with previous reports indicating that TD in older patients seems to be more persistent than in younger patients (34, 35).

Apart from a longer stay in hospital in TD patients, which may reflect severity of illness, no single factor has been implicated in the development of this side effect. Several studies had indicated that TD may develop in family members who are treated with neuroleptics (36, 37). Thus variations in individual susceptibility, which may be linked to genetic factors, may be of importance in the development of TD and deserve extensive investigation.

REFERENCES

1 Schonecker M: Ein eigentum biches Syndrom in oralen Bereich bei Megaphen. Applikation Nervenarzt 28:35, 1957

2. Kane JM, Smith JM: Tardive dyskinesia: prevalence and risk factors, 1959 to 1979. Arch Gen Psychiatry 59:473–481, 1982

3. Brandon S, McClelland HA, Protheroe C: A study of facial dyskinesia in a mental hospital population. Br J Psychiatry 118:171–184, 1971

4. Jeste DV, Wyatt RJ: Understanding and treating tardive dyskinesia. J Clin Psychiatry 46 (Suppl 4):14–18, 1985

5. Yassa R, Nair NPV: Incidence of tardive dyskinesia in an outpatient population. Psychosomatics 25:479–481, 1984

6. Wolf ME, Ryan JJ, Mosnaim AD: Organicity and tardive dyskinesia. Psychosomatics 23:475–480, 1982

7. Jeste DV, Wyatt RJ: Prevention and Management of Tardive Dyskinesia. New York, Guilford Press, 1982

8. Jeste DV, Potkin SG, Sinha S, et al: Tardive dyskinesia: reversible and persistent. Arch Gen Psychiatry 36:585–590, 1979

9. Yassa R, Ghadirian AM, Schwartz G: Tardive dyskinesia: developmental factors. Can J Psychiatry 30:344–347, 1985

10. Yassa R, Nair V, Schwartz G: Tardive dyskinesia and the primary psychiatric diagnosis. Psychosomatics 25:135–138, 1984

11. Yassa R, Nair V, Schwartz G: Early versus late onset psychosis and tardive dyskinesia. Biol Psychiatry 21:1291–1297, 1980

12. Rosennbaum AH, Niven RG, Hanson NP: Tardive dyskinesia: relationship with a primary affective disorder. Dis Nerv Syst 38:423–427, 1977

13. Yassa R, Ghadirian AM, Schwartz G: Prevalence of tardive dyskinesia in affective disorder patients. J Clin Psychiatry 43:410–412, 1983

14. Wolf ME, DeWolfe AS, Ryan JJ, et al: Vulnerability to tardive dyskinesia. J. Clin Psychiatry 46:367–368, 1985

15. Jus A, Pineau R, Lachance R, et al: Epidemiology of tardive dyskinesia: Part II. Dis Nerv Syst 37:257–261, 1976

16. Chouinard G, Ross-Chouinard A: Factors related to tardive dyskinesia. Am J Psychiatry 136:79–83, 1979

17. Perenyi A, Arato M: Tardive dyskinesia on Hungarian psychiatric wards. Psychosomatics 21:904–909, 1980

18. Jeste DV, Kleinman JE, Potkin SG, et al: Ex Uno Multi: subtyping the schizophrenic syndrome. Biol Psychiatry 17:199–222, 1982

19. Demars JP: Neuromuscular effects of long-term phenothiazine medication, electroconvulsive therapy and leucotomy. J Nerv Ment Dis 113:73–79, 1966

20. Siede H, Muller HF: Choreiform movements as side effects of phenothiazine medication in geriatric patients. J Am Geriatr Soc 15:517–522, 1967

21. Greenblatt DL, Dominick JR, Stotsky BA, et al: Phenothiazine-induced dyskinesia in nursing-home patients. J Am Geriatr Soc 16:27–31, 1968

22. Crane GE, Smeets RA: Tardive dyskinesia and drug therapy in geriatric patients. Arch Gen Psychiatry 30:341–343, 1973

23. Bourgeois M, Bouille P, Tignol Y, et al: Spontaneous dyskinesias vs neuroleptic-induced dyskinesias in 270 elderly subjects. J Nerv Ment Dis 168:177–178, 1974

24. Delwaide PJ, Desseilles M: Spontaneous buccolinguofacial dyskinesia in the elderly. Acta Neurol Scand 56:256–262, 1977

25. Kane JM, Weinhold P, Kinon B: Prevalence of abnormal involuntary movements in the normal elderly. Psychopharmacology 77:105–108, 1982

26. Klawans HL, Barr A: Prevalence of spontaneous lingual facial buccal dyskinesias in the elderly. Neurology 32:558–559, 1982

27. Varga E, Sugerman AA, Varga V, et al: Prevalence of spontaneous oral dyskinesia in the elderly. Am J Psychiatry 139:329–331, 1982

28. Lieberman J, Kane JM, Woerner M, et al: Prevalence of tardive dyskinesia in elderly patients. Psychopharmacol Bull 20:22–26, 1985

29. Toenniessen LM, Casey DE, MacFarland BH: Tardive dyskinesia in the aged: duration of treatment relationships. Arch Gen Psychiatry 42:278–284, 1985

30. Chorfi M, Moussaoui D: Les schizophrenes jamais traites n'ont pas de movements anormaux type diskinesie tardive. L'Encephale II: 263–265, 1985

31. Kane JM, Woerner M, Lieberman JA, et al: Tardive dyskinesias and drugs. Drug Development Research 9:41–51, 1986

32. Cunningham-Owens DG, Johnstone EC, Frith CD: Spontaneous involuntary disorders of movement: their prevalence, severity and distribution in chronic schizophrenics with and without treatment with neuroleptics. Arch Gen Psychiatry 39:452–461, 1982

33. Crow TJ, Cross AJ, Johnstone EC, et al: Abnormal involuntary movements in schizophrenia: are they related to the disease process or its treatment? Are they associated with changes in dopamine receptors? J Clin Psychopharmacol 2:336–340, 1982

34. Smith JM, Baldessarini RJ: Changes in prevalence, severity and recovery in tardive dyskinesia with age. Arch Gen Psychiatry 37:1368–1373, 1980

35. Yassa R, Nair V, Schwartz G: Tardive dyskinesia: a two-year followup study. Psychosomatics 25:852–855, 1984b

36. Weinhold P, Wegner JT, Kane JM: Familial occurrence of tardive dyskinesia. J Clin Psychiatry 42:165–166, 1981

37. Yassa R, Ananth J: Familial tardive dyskinesia. Am J Psychiatry 138:1618–1619, 1981

Chapter 10

Tardive Dyskinesia in Special Populations

C. Thomas Gualtieri, M.D.
L. Jarrett Barnhill, M.D.

Chapter 10

Tardive Dyskinesia in Special Populations

Aremarkable change has taken place in the past 10 years, a change that coincides with physicians' growing concern over the problem of tardive dyskinesia (TD). The prescription of neuroleptic drugs had declined markedly for mentally retarded patients and child psychiatry patients. At one time, not long ago, neuroleptics like thioridazine and haloperidol were widely prescribed to children who were hyperactive or emotionally unstable; neuroleptics were virtually the only psychotropic prescribed for retarded people with any behavior problem at all. This practice seems to have changed. Neuroleptic treatment is considered by enlightened practitioners in the field to be an extraordinary intervention, one that is not to be undertaken for mild disorders where other treatments may be more effective. For children, the only acceptable indications are schizophrenia and severe cases of Tourette's syndrome (TS) (1). For retarded people, the only accepted indications are schizophrenia, TS, and some severe cases of self-injurious behavior (2, 3).

The reasons for this change of view are:

1. The realization that only limited therapeutic success is to be gained from neuroleptic prescription in these populations;
2. The discovery of intelligent alternatives to neuroleptics—the psychotropic anticonvulsants, calcium channel blockers, beta-blockers, and lithium; and
3. The discovery of high rates of TD in these patient groups (3).

A third group of patients, victims of closed head injury (CHI) with "neurobehavioral sequelae" are a relatively new patient population. In contrast to child psychiatry and mental retardation, the field of CHI does not have a history of neuroleptic overuse; the prevailing attitude in that young and emerging field has always been one of "therapeutic nihilism"—emphasizing rehabilitation, deemphasizing pharmacology. CHI patients represent a third group for whom neuroleptics are "relatively contraindicated" (4).

TARDIVE DYSKINESIA IN CHILDREN

Anecdotal reports of neuroleptic-induced movement disorders have appeared in the literature for quite some time (5, 6). Systematic investigations concerned with the epidemiology and course of TD in children are a more recent phenomena, however (7). The reasons for this delayed interest are myriad, derived perhaps from the notion that children were relatively safe from irreversible neuroleptic effects (8); that small neuroleptic doses posed few risks; or that in severe psychiatric disease, no alternative treatments were available or considered. The present application of TD as a public health problem has helped to revise this attitude.

Clinical investigations of TD follow a predictable trend. Early studies focused on case descriptions, and then came studies of incidence and prevalence. Subsequent epidemiologic work focuses on prevention and reducing morbidity. Prevention studies try to define at-risk populations; try to solidify diagnostic processes and the justification for neuroleptic treatment; emphasize trial drug withdrawals and low-dose treatment techniques; and try to find alternatives to neuroleptic treatment. The development of sophisticated "at risk" strategies and of alternative treatment approaches has been complicated in child psychiatry by relative weakness of neuropsychiatric research in the field. Relative unawareness of advances in biological and psychopharmacological treatments by child psychiatrists and pediatricians has probably compounded the problem of TD in this population.

Part of the difficulty, however, lies in the complexity of TD. Attempts to map the pathophysiology of TD have yielded ambiguous results. Neuroleptic-induced dopaminergic supersensitivity is too simple a model and fails to explain the existence of persistent dyskinesia. Other ambiguous factors include the varying effects of cholinergic drugs, the occasional favorable responses to dopamine agonists (9), and inconsistent results from attempts to manipulate the gamma-aminobutyric (GABA) receptor (10).

In addition, the variability of dyskinetic movements in response to manipulation of neuroleptics confounds the issue. Breakthrough dyskinesias seem different from withdrawal dyskinesias, mainly in terms of persistence and perhaps severity (5, 7, 11). In children, the unanswered question is why there is a preponderance of withdrawal or transient dyskinesias relative to the incidence of persistent dyskinesias. The simplest explanation is that cumulative exposure in children is rarely sufficient to induce a persistent TD syndrome. But that is only a hypothetical explanation. The possibility of an interaction between age and neuroleptic toxicity cannot be discounted; such an interaction would also explain why, at the other end of the spectrum, elderly people appear to be more vulnerable to severe and persistent TD.

The description of childhood TD has undergone an evolution. The repertoire of movements was initially described as more centrifugal in distribution, involving predominantly peripheral dystonic and choreiform-like movements (12). With greater systematic experience, this topographical distribution has been modified to overlap the pattern of adult TD (5, 7).

Various neurochemical studies of childhood psychopathology intimate a high incidence of dopaminergic dysfunction (11, 13). The introduction of neuroleptics may not only affect immediate risks but potential, long-term maturational changes. Reduced serum estrogen levels in prepubertal children may also have some undefined effect on dopamine neurotransmission and receptor sensitivity (14).

One additional question remains unanswered. What are the long-term effects of disruption of neurotransmittor systems in the maturing organism? Does the fact that TD in children is usually transient actually mean that they have really escaped a debilitating disorder? The question is whether early neuroleptic exposure may lead to a latent weakness in dopamine systems such that degenerative changes will appear in later years. Precedents exist: kindling effects in temporal lobe epilepsy, postpoliomyelitis deterioration, postencephalitic Parkinson's disease, and late-onset psychosis following CHI.

TD in the Mentally Retarded

Although neuroleptics are commonly prescribed for developmentally disabled patients, they are usually misapplied. Most surveys of large populations have revealed similar findings:

1. Neuroleptic use ranges from 19 percent to roughly 25 percent of institutional and community-based patients. Ten years ago the rate was about 50 percent (2).
2. Most patients lack a clear psychiatric diagnosis (less than 6 percent in institutions, less than 3 percent in community settings (15, 16).
3. Many patients are treated with relatively large doses or in situations involving polypharmacy (15, 17, 18).

4. Many treatment programs are carried on for extended periods of time without careful monitoring (3, 5, 17, 18).

These practices have created a large pool of patients who are at high risk for TD. On the basis of available data, rates for TD may exceed 34 percent of patients on chronic neuroleptic treatments (3, 5). This figure falls within the ranges associated with neuroleptic treatment in nonhandicapped psychiatric populations (19). It is not clear whether severe or persistent dyskinesias are more common in the developmentally disabled.

Several risk factors may be involved in the development of TD in the developmentally disabled. At this point, total cumulative dose appears to correlate most clearly with the emergency of TD (3, 7, 10). The prescribing patterns noted earlier may surely heighten this factor. A higher incidence of encephalopathy associated with severe developmental disorders may also influence vulnerability (3, 20).

The retarded population displays an increased rate of behavioral abnormalities such as hyperactivity, aggression, self-injurious behavior, and stereotypies, as well as high rate of institutionalization. It is likely that rates of neuroleptic treatment are high, especially by poorly trained physicians who do not appreciate the availability of alternative treatments. In many of these clinical situations, neuroleptics have been considered front-line treatment (17).

As the level of intellectual function and communication skills diminishes, the reliability of psychiatric diagnoses tends to follow suit (21). Low IQ may also affect a physician's assessment of emerging extrapyramidal symptoms, in particular, akathisia. A patient's poor verbal skills combined with an unusual akathisia may prompt the unwitting physician to increase the neuroleptic dose. Such a pharmacologic tail-chase will only increase the patient's eventual risk of developing TD by guaranteeing continued neuroleptic use at increasing doses, while potential warning signs of TD are suppressed. More troublesome is the relative lack of reported breakthrough dyskinesias on maintenance neuroleptics (3). These emergent symptoms (particularly vermicular tongue movements and choreiform hand movements) alert clinicians to the presence of TD. Such harbinger symptoms may signal the need to reduce or to discontinue neuroleptics and presumably reduce the risk for more severe persistent dyskinesia. Lacking this signal, clinicians must episodically reduce the dose of neuroleptics. Even with this approach, dyskinetic movements may emerge only after a lag of between 1 to 4 weeks (3, 7). The mentally retarded patient may have some difficulty tolerating this lag. Many patients will show significant behavior deterioration off the drug, even if it has not been particularly beneficial in the first place, with dramatic increases in premedication behaviors, or the emergence of new "rebound" symptoms (3, 22–24). This vulnerability requires special strategies for management, intense environmental structure, behavioral management, and sometimes the resumption of the offending neuroleptic drug.

COURSE OF TARDIVE DYSKINESIA IN MENTALLY RETARDED ADULTS

A more critical concern, once tardive dyskinesia has been diagnosed, is the course of tardive dyskinesia in individuals who continue on neuroleptic treatment.

Does the resumption of neuroleptic treatment necessarily mean that the disorder will grow worse, or is the course of the disorder variable or idiosyncratic? The literature is silent on this point, since most tardive dyskinesia research has been done in patients examined at a single point in time. Further, if neuroleptic withdrawal is not a part of a patient evaluation for tardive dyskinesia, the masking effect of maintenance neuroleptic treatment may obscure the proper assessment of severity of dyskinesia. The only prospective longitudinal study of tardive dyskinesia of which the authors are aware has not yet gathered data sufficient to address the question of course (25). In one study of TD patients maintained off neuroleptics, no appreciable symptom reduction was noted after 12 months, and the authors concluded that the disorder is for the most part unremitting (26). This is at variance with clinical experience that seems to suggest that improvement in symptoms of TD may sometimes occur, even years after the disorder is originally diagnosed. There is one study from a Danish sample, not yet published, that suggests that TD may remit even in patients who continue a neuroleptic treatment (D. Casey, personal communication, 1984). In a 2-year follow-up study by Yassa, Nair, and Schwartz (27), most TD patients (66 percent) showed no change, while equal proportions improved (18 percent) or worsened (16 percent). However, neuroleptic masking effects may compromise this finding. Paulson, Rizvi, and Crane (28) reexamined institutionalized retarded children 4 years after an original drug withdrawal trial and found no change in TD in six children; four displayed more severe dyskinesias, and five had improved. However, the patients' medication status in the interval between observations and during the follow-up period was not stated.

One aspect of our research was to measure the occurrence of dyskinetic movements during a second neuroleptic drug withdrawal in 12 mentally retarded individuals who had been involved in a similar withdrawal 3 years previously (7). It was hypothesized that the severity of dyskinetic movements in the second withdrawal would increase following continued treatment and would be associated with each subject's increment in lifetime cumulative dose of neuroleptic drug.

Subjects were eight male and four female profoundly retarded, long-term residents of a state mental retardation facility who had participated in a previous study (7). The 12 residents were on the average 30.7 years old (range = 22–41 years), had mean IQs of 11 (range = 10–23) and mean Vineland Social Quotients of 10.2 (range = 4–25). All subjects had a continuous, lengthy neuroleptic history prior to the original study and did not have other conditions (for example, cerebral palsy) which might produce abnormal involuntary movements. At the start of the original and the present studies respectively, 12 of 12 and 8 of 12 subjects were receiving neuroleptic medication. Each resident's cumulative neuroleptic history before the first study and average daily dose in a comparable period before each study is presented in Table 1. The medications were prescribed for aberrant behaviors such as aggression, self-injury, property destruction, or noncompliance. Each subject lived in a 24-hour residential treatment unit with 15 to 25 similarly functioning individuals and received several hours of adaptive skill training each day. Prior to the second withdrawal, four subjects were receiving thioridazine, three haloperidol, one thiothixene, and four not any psychoactive medication at all. All subjects were healthy and on no intercurrent medication.

Three psychologists rated location and severity of dyskinetic movements using the Abnormal Involuntary Movement Scale (AIMS) (29). Raters were trained in a fashion similar to a previous study, using videotapes, "live" observation of individuals with dyskinetic movements, and discussion of practice ratings to clarify disagreements. Practice ratings continued until all three observers independently and simultaneously agreed on the specific location of each subject's dyskinetic movements with no difference greater than one unit of severity (none, minimal, mild, moderate, severe). Reliability was also checked with a rater (the first author) who had conducted examinations in the original study (7). The four raters agreed on location and severity of 93 percent of items with a difference of 1 or less and the remaining 7 percent of items showed a difference of 2. The three psychologists showed agreement in this observation similar to that initially established.

During each weekly examination, the rater and the subject were alone in a quiet room. The AIMS examination procedure (29) was followed as closely as the adaptive level of the subject permitted. Raters were assigned randomly to observe subjects each week and were not aware of any subject's current or past medication status. After a variable baseline, subjects were withdrawn from medication in a double-blind fashion. After withdrawal subjects were off med-

Table 1. Occurrence of Dyskinetic Movements During a Second Neuroleptic Drug Withdrawal in 12 Mentally Retarded Individuals

Group, subject	Sex	Cumulative dose before first study[a] (g)	Mean daily dose at withdrawal (mg)	Mean total AIMS score
Group 1: Medication increased				
2	F	5,804	a. 1,000	a. 2.2
			b. 2,750	b. 7.0
3	M	562	a. 75	a. 0.6
			b. 200	b. 5.0
7	F	4,177	a. 150	a. 2.8
			b. 190	b. 4.0
11	M	62	a. 75	a. 0.0
			b. 237	b. 0.9
Group 2: Medication decreased				
1	M	3,956	a. 60	a. 17.8
			b. 40	b. 11.1
8	F	3,474	a. 300	a. 7.3
			b. 130	b. 4.5
10	M	1,133	a. 225	a. 0.6
			b. 137	b. 0.0
12	F	3,209	a. 750	a. 12.4
			b. 683	b. 4.0
Group 3: Medication discontinued				
4	M	45	a. 50	a. 0.0
			b. 0	b. 0.1
5	M	11,188	a. 300	a. 7.5
			b. 0	b. 5.5
6	M	316	a. 150	a. 0.0
			b. 0	b. 1.2
9	F	160	a. 75	a. 0.0
			b. 0	b. 0.0

Note. AIMS—Abnormal Involuntary Movement Scale. a. = first withdrawal. b. = second withdrawal.

[a]Chlorpromazine equivalent.

ication from 1 to 15 weeks. Subjects 10 and 11 were not withdrawn from medication because of staff concerns about aberrant behavior. The criteria for diagnosing TD were those recommended by Gualtieri et al (30). Three additional cases of TD were noted in the second withdrawal (Subjects 3, 6, and 11) in addition to the six cases reported in the original trial (Subjects 1, 2, 5, 7, 8, and 12). Five subjects (2, 3, 6, 7, and 11) displayed more severe dyskinetic movements after the second withdrawal. These subjects, except for Subject 6, received neuroleptics at a mean daily oral dose greater than a similar period prior to the first withdrawal (see Table 1). Subject 6 was not returned to a neuroleptic after the first withdrawal but showed a small increase in dyskinetic movements. Four subjects (1, 5, 8, and 12) displayed less severe movements during the second withdrawal; these individuals received lower doses of neuroleptic medication between studies. Three subjects (4, 9, and 10) did not display dyskinetic movements in either withdrawal trial.

These withdrawal data were categorized into three groups based on neuroleptic status between studies: medication increased (Group 1), decreased (Group 2), and discontinued (Group 3). Mean total AIMS data were analyzed using a 3×2 analysis of coveriance (Group $\times$ Trial) with cumulative lifetime neuroleptic dose prior to the first withdrawal as the covariate. This analysis, which was statistically controlled for cumulative dose, was not significant for main group effects but yielded the following for the interaction terms: $F(2, 8) = 3.81$, $p < .07$. A post-hoc Newman-Keuls analysis revealed significant differences for the following comparisons: Group 2, Trial 1 versus Group 1, Trial 1 ($p < .01$); Group 2, Trial 1 versus Group 1, Trial 2 ($p < .05$); Group 2, Trial 1 versus Group 3, Trial 1 ($p < .05$); Group 2, Trial 1 versus Group 3, Trial 2 ($p < .01$); and Group 2, Trial 1 versus Group 2, Trial 2 ($p < .05$). Salient aspects of the Newman-Keuls comparisons are as follows: 1) Group 2, the individuals with the highest cumulative neuroleptic history, had significantly more severe dyskinetic movements than Groups 1 or 3 during the first trial. 2) Group 2 showed a significant decrease in severity of movements between withdrawal trials. 3) Differences between groups during the second withdrawal trial were nonsignificant. And 4) Group 1 was the only group that showed an increase between trials in severity of dyskinesia with a trend toward statistical significance.

The results of this second withdrawal trial indicated that 9 of 12 individuals met the tardive dyskinesia movement criteria, 3 more than in the first trial. Within-subject comparisons revealed that five subjects displayed more severe movements, four subjects displayed movements that were less severe, and three subjects did not display any dyskinetic movements in the second or in the first withdrawal trial.

One may draw the following conclusions from these results. First, dyskinetic movements may persist over time regardless of change in neuroleptic status. This was evident in all seven subjects who were returned to a neuroleptic after the first withdrawal study. Subjects 5 and 6 who displayed dyskinesias in the first withdrawal and were not returned to a neuroleptic still showed movements in the second study. These results replicate the frequently reported finding that neuroleptic-induced dyskinesias persist over time (31). Second, severity of dyskinetic movements may change over time in the same direction as the increase or decrease of neuroleptic dosage, independent of prior cumulative exposure. Group 1 subjects, with the lowest prestudy 1 cumulative dose history, received increased dosages of neuroleptics between studies and were the only group to show an increase in the severity of dyskinetic movements. Subjects in Group 2 received lower doses of neuroleptics between studies and showed a decrease in severity of movements. While these results do not necessarily contradict the importance of lifetime cumulative dose as predictor for occurrence of tardive dyskinesia (7, 31), the data do suggest that severity of dyskinetic movements at a specific point in time may be related more to the recent history of neuroleptic dose rather than to a lifetime exposure or duration of treatment. They represent indirect support of a dopamine supersensitivity hypothesis of TD (10).

It is not possible to draw strong conclusions from a study of only 12 patients. Further, data from mentally retarded patients may not be generalized to patients of normal intelligence; the prevalence of TD, its severity, and perhaps also its course may be more problematic in the former group (7). This application of a serial neuroleptic withdrawal method is unique in the TD literature, however, and demands careful attention. TD may not remit spontaneously in retarded patients, and continued treatment, especially with high doses, may make it worse. On the other hand, if continued neuroleptic treatment is necessary, the application of low doses may prevent the aggravation of TD.

WHY NEUROLEPTIC USE SHOULD BE AVOIDED IN CLOSED HEAD INJURY

Each year, there are more than 800,000 serious cases of CHI in the United States. Ninety percent of the victims survive their injury (only 10 percent survived 10 years ago). Fifty to ninety thousand people suffer injuries that leave severe residual symptoms or deficits. Since the majority of CHI victims are young (peak incidence is between ages 18 and 24), the cumulative number of such patients will continue to rise, year by year, for a long time to come. (Figures are from the National Head Injury Foundation.)

Even mild head injuries may result in significant symptoms: the so-called "post-concussive syndrome." Many mild head injuries are never reported. Most physicians fail to relate psychological problems to a mild head injury; the tendency, then, is to underestimate the extent of the problem. The actual number of CHI patients is probably much higher than we have ever believed.

Brain injury will necessarily lead to a wide range of symptoms and deficits. As a general rule, the severity of the injury will determine the severity of outcome. Some of the problems of CHI patients are attributable to the specific focus of damage. More commonly, however, residual problems are the consequence of diffuse cortical damage or of damage to axial brain structures that modulate cortical function. Since anterior, frontal, and temporal lobe structures are most frequently damaged in CHI, many of the sequelae are referable to these structures. It is believed that the shear forces that damage axial or subcortical structures in CHI are probably responsible for problems in memory, attention, emotional regulation, and arousal (32, 33). It is this combination of specific cortical damage and diffuse subcortical damage that renders the CHI patient a unique specimen.

Advocates insist that the clinical needs of CHI patients are different from those of other patients, and in this contention they are probably correct. CHI patients are not like stroke patients, or developmentally handicapped patients, or psychiatric patients; they are different, and unique. Physicians and therapists who were originally trained with other patient groups soon discover that major adjustments in therapeutic approach are necessary when the sequelae of CHI are at issue. So it is, too, when pharmacological approaches are brought to bear.

The following is a typical neuroleptic scenario for CHI patients: A patient is treated with intramuscular and then with oral haloperidol, to control agitation and assaultiveness during emergence from coma. The drug is almost inadvertently continued for months after discharge from the hospital. Then the patient appears for evaluation at a rehabilitation facility, anergic, depressed, and apathetic, with fine and gross motor coordination problems and deficits in attention, memory, and emotional control. The neuroleptic is withdrawn, and there is immediate improvement in all of these areas.

This is a typical example of short-term benefit for an appropriate indication—acute agitation—turning into inappropriate long-term treatment. The more intelligent course would have been to gradually taper the neuroleptic after the patient's emotional state was stable for a couple of weeks. Neuroleptics should usually be tapered, not withdrawn abruptly. Abrupt withdrawal from neuroleptics may precipitate seizures (34); abrupt withdrawal can also be the occasion for prompt relapse with severe behavior problems. Stepwise reduction by 25 percent decrements over 4 weeks usually averts such problems.

Agitation, explosiveness, emotional instability, disorganization, and psychosis in CHI patients are not necessarily confined to the immediate post-recovery period. They may be persistent symptoms of CHI. In such instances, neuroleptics may be indicated, although they may not always be effective. Relatively short trials of two or three neuroleptics, in succession, ought to be sufficient to determine whether treatment is going to be successful, and if it is not successful, it is common sense to withdraw the patient from neuroleptics, reestablish a baseline, and try some other approach. Low to moderate doses are usually sufficient to establish whether a neuroleptic will be useful. High-dose treatment is rarely, if ever, necessary. It seems trite to warn against long-term treatment with an ineffective medication, but with neuroleptics, the pattern is too common to ignore.

Tourette's syndrome may be the consequence of CHI, and low-dose neuroleptics are occasionally helpful. Low dose neuroleptics may actually enhance cognitive performance, for example, in attentional tasks (7), probably a presynaptic stimulant-like effect (3).

Low-potency neuroleptics like thioridazine (Mellaril) and chlorpromazine (Thorazine) tend to be sedating, and thioridazine in particular is a strongly anticholinergic neuroleptic. It also appears that the neuroleptic chlorpromazine may impair short-term memory at doses below those required to cause motor impairment (35). Such drugs probably should be avoided in CHI patients. The high-potency neuroleptics are less sedating and are preferred when a neuroleptic is required. Representatives of this class include fluphenazine (Prolixin), trifluoperazine (Stelazine), and haloperidol (Haldol). Haloperidol commonly causes dysphoria, however. High-potency neuroleptics are more likely to cause acute extrapyramidal reactions and the neuroleptic malignant syndrome.

Neuroleptics can lower the seizure threshold. Pimozide and fluphenazine are two neuroleptics least likely to do so. Haloperidol and thioridazine are among the most likely to lower the seizure threshold (34, 36).

Do neuroleptics compromise the recovery process for CHI patients? Yes, if one extrapolates from the preclinical studies and from human studies of neuroleptic-induced anhedonia (37), dysphoria (38), and cognitive and motor impairment (39). Yes, indeed, if one is guided by the prevailing belief that deficits in dopaminergic neurotransmission are central to the pathophysiology of CHI. One is thus inclined to consider neuroleptics relatively contraindicated in CHI patients, except for those subjects with neuroleptic-responsive psychosis, hallucinosis, mania, Tourette's syndrome, assaultiveness, or agitation. The key is to determine whether the symptoms are indeed "neuroleptic responsive," that is, that the drugs exert dramatic clinical effects when no other treatment will work as well; that their efficacy is established at a "minimal effective dose"; and that their continued clinical utility is assessed at reasonable intervals, say, every 6 months, by gradually tapering the dose. There is nothing "rational" about long-term large-dose neuroleptic treatment for CHI patients.

The issue is not only even the negative cognitive or motor effects of neuroleptics, or their tendency to "blunt" the personality of treated patients. It is only in small part influenced by their serious side effects: dysphoria, pseudo-parkinsonism, dystonia, tardive dyskinesia, hyperthermia, and the "neuroleptic malignant syndrome," photosensitivity, cholestatic jaundice, hypotension. It is in its largest dimensions defined by their limited utility in the long-term management of CHI patients, and the superior effects to be won by more carefully selected psychotropic treatments. Neuroleptics may be the best and only drug treatment for schizophrenia, but they are usually a poor third to carbamazepine and lithium for patients whose symptoms are a consequence of "organic" brain disorder.

Preexisting brain damage is sometimes listed as a risk factor for tardive dyskinesia. The clinical evidence is equivocal on this point, but the research is suggestive (40). Long-term neuroleptic treatment in CHI patients requires careful monitoring for TD.

A Behavioral Analog of TD

The question of a behavioral "analog" of TD is a good example of the limitations of inferential research. The idea is that chronic neuroleptic treatment may also afflict "higher" areas of brain and that dementia, psychosis, and/or emotional instability may be the consequence of suprastriatal neuroleptic effects. Terms like "supersensitivity psychosis" and "tardive dysmentia" have been coined to capture the phenomenon, and there are animal models of postsynaptic receptor supersensitivity in the mesolimbic dopamine system. The notion is not supported by any direct evidence; it is only a surmise based on indirect evidence.

The fundamental problem is how to demonstrate a connection

between neuroleptics and cortical dysfunction when cortical dysfunction of one sort or another characterizes a large proportion of the patients who are treated with neuroleptics to begin with. How can one draw inferences based on the expected natural history of neuroleptic-treated patients when the conditions for which drugs are most commonly prescribed are known to have an extremely variable course, and when the patients are often compelled to spend their lives in degrading circumstances that may of themselves lead to psychological deterioration? Even were one to demonstrate dopamine receptor proliferation in human brains, in frontal cortex or the limbic system, the natural question would be whether this was the consequence of the drugs or of the primary disease that afflicted the patient. There is no clearer demonstration of the limitations of TD research than this; if one cannot cultivate a no-treatment control group, the definitive answer will always be elusive.

There are several alternative strategies that may be mounted to deal with the question. Considering the alternative approaches is an interesting lesson in the scientific method.

Alternative 1 is to ignore the problem. After all, it is a hard question to test, and any result will be contested anyway. There are other research priorities.

This is not a bad idea. After all, the demonstration of a "higher" neuroleptic effect should not enjoin practitioners to greater caution with respect to neuroleptic treatment than they currently exercise in the face of TD or the neuroleptic malignant syndrome.

However, there is a problem with alternative 1: We miss an opportunity to surmount a scientific challenge simply because it is difficult. We lose an opportunity to learn how neuroleptics affect the dynamics of neural systems. These might be theoretical questions today, but they may have practical importance years hence, when antipsychotics that do not work on striatal receptors are developed, and the need to measure their long-term psychological impact is upon us.

Alternative 2 is to assume that neuroleptics do affect higher cortical centers. After all, why shouldn't they? Simply place the burden of proof on those who maintain that neuroleptics have no long-term psychological effects. This is not an extreme position. In virtually every clinical survey that has addressed the question, it is found that TD patients, compared to non-TD patients, have more in the way of dementia (41). It is the interpretation of these data that is at issue—whether one presumes that the neuroleptic caused dementia, or that dementia predisposed patients treated with neuroleptics to develop TD, or that some kind of interaction is operating. Is there a reason to suppose that one interpretation is preferred? It is our opinion that the first interpretation is not tenable and that the truth of the matter probably rests with the second or the third. The reasoning behind this opinion is as follows: Patients with "organic" brain disease have not been shown to be at greater risk for TD than patients with "functional" disorders. The prevalence of TD in retarded people is probably no higher than in schizophrenic patients (1, 3). In contrast, patients with affective disorders may be at greater risk to develop TD than any other clinical group (42, 43).

The high prevalence of persistent TD in elderly populations suggests an interaction between antipsychotic drug neurotoxicity and some pharmacodynamic elements intrinsic in the aging process (8).

Persistent TD is probably the consequence of irreversible striatal damage. But the corpus striatum is responsible for more than motor control; it is a complex organ that influences a wide range of complex human behaviors (44, 45). No disease that afflicts striatal tissue is known to have only motor consequences; Parkinson's disease and Huntington's diesease are only two examples.

This approach sidesteps the issue of mesocortical and mesolimbic damage and emphasizes the psychological importance of striatal damage. It is an interesting approach because it generates a testable hypothesis: that TD patients, compared to non-TD patients, will have specific neuropsychological impairment in tests known to be sensitive to striatal lesions, delayed response, for example (46). A research strategy like this will only be effective, however, if it is linked to a prospective study design. If the hypothesis were tested in a design that identified patients in a point-prevalence survey, there would be no way of distinguishing between drug-induced striatal effects of predrug deficits in striatal function that predisposed patients to the development of TD.

It is likely that the best way to approach the question of whether dopamine receptor proliferation in human brains is the consequence of the drug or the primary disease will be to look for specific psychological or behavioral changes in primates treated with long-term neuroleptics. Here the research is simplified considerably by the possibility of comparing neuroleptic-treated animals to untreated controls. If a specific behavioral syndrome were to be demonstrated in primates with TD, then the model of that syndrome could be investigated in humans with and without TD. The strategy is still indirect, but less so than strategies relying exclusively on human populations.

The lesson of science is that as simple questions are addressed, more complicated questions arise. Scientists only succeed, it seems, in making work for new generations of scientists. As we begin to acquire some fundamental epidemiological information about TD, we are left with the imperative to advance our knowledge in areas that are less explicit and more complex. As we master the methods to study the epidemiology of TD, we are left with the challenge of untangling the neuropsychology of the disorder.

REFERENCES

1. American Psychiatric Association Task Force Report on Tardive Dyskinesia: Washington, DC, American Psychiatric Association, in press

2. Gualtieri CT: Pharmacotherapy and neurobehavioral sequelae of traumatic brain injury. Brain Injury, in press

3. Gualtieri CT, Schroeder SR, Hicks, et al: Tardive dyskinesia in young mentally retarded individuals. Arch Gen Psychiatry 43:335–340, 1986

4. Gualtieri CT: Mental retardation, in Treatments of Psychiatric Disorders: A Task Force Report of the American Psychiatric Association. Washington, DC, American Psychiatric Association, in press

5. Gualtieri CT, Barnhill J, McGimsey J, et al: Tardive dyskinesia and other movement disorders in children. Am Acad Child Psychiatry 19:491–510, 1980

6. Polizos P, Engelhardt D: Dyskinetic and neuroleptic complications in children treated with psychotropic medication, in Tardive Dyskinesia: Research and Treatment. Edited by Fann WE, Smith RC, Davis JM, et al. Jamaica, NY, Spectrum Press, 1980, pp. 193–199

7. Gualtieri CT, Quade D, Hicks RE, et al: Tardive dyskinesia and other consequences of neuroleptic treatment in children and adolescents. Am J Psychiatry 141:20–23, 1984

8. Smith JM, Baldessarini RJ: Changes in prevalence and severity of TD with age. Arch Gen Psychiatry 37:1368–1373, 1980

9. Carrol BK, Curtis GC: Paradoxical response to dopamine agonists in tardive dyskinesia. Am J Psychiatry 134:785–789, 1977

10. Baldessarini RJ, Tarsy O: Tardive dyskinesia, in Psychopharmacology: A Generation of Progress. Edited by DiMascio A, Killam KR. New York, Raven Press, 1978, pp. 993–1004

11. Teicher MR, Baldessarini RJ: Developmental pharmacokinetics, in Psychiatric Pharmacokinetics of Children and Adolescents. Edited by Pepper C. Washington, DC, American Psychiatric Press, 1987, pp. 45–80

12. Engelhardt DM, Polizos P, Waizer J: Consequence of psychotropic drug withdrawal in autistic children: A follow-up study. Psychopharmacol Bull 11:6–7, 1975

13. Coyle J: Biochemical development of the brain and neurotransmitters in child psychiatry, in Psychiatric Pharmacokinetics of Children and Adolescents. Edited by Pepper C. Washington, DC, American Psychiatric Press, 1987, pp. 1–26

14. Villeneuve A, Cazejust T, Cote M: Estrogens and tardive dyskinesia in male psychiatric patients. Neuropsychobiology 6:145–151, 1980

15. Hill BK, Barlow EA, Bruininks RH: A national study of prescribed drugs in institution and community residential facilities for mentally retarded people. Psychopharmacol Bull 21:279–284, 1985

16. Intagliata J, Rinek C: Psychoactive drug use in public and community residential facilities for mentally retarded people. Psychopharmacol Bull 20:268–278, 1985

17. Lipman RS, DiMascio A: Psychotropic drugs and mentally retarded children, in Psychopharmacology: A Generation of Progress. Edited by Lipton MA, DiMascio A, Killam KR. New York, Raven Press, 1978, pp. 1437–1449

18. Sprague RL: Overview of psychopharmacology for the retarded in the U.S., in Research to Practice in MR: Biomedical Aspects. Edited by Mittler P. Baltimore, MD, University Park Press, 1977, pp. 199–202

19. Kane JA, Woerner M, Liberman J, et al: Tardive dyskinesia, in Neuropsychiatry of Movement Disorders. Edited by Jeste DV, Wyatt RJ. Washington, DC, American Psychiatric Press, 1984, pp. 97–118

20. Kaufman CA, Jeste DV, Shelton RC, et al: Noradrenergic and neuroradiological abnormalities in tardive dyskinesia. Biol Psychiatry 21:781–799, 1986

21. Menolascino FJ, Levitas A, Greiner C: Nature and types of mental illness in the mentally retarded. Psychopharmacol Bull 22:1060–1067, 1986

22. Gualtieri CT, Hawk B: TD and other drug-induced movement disorders among handicapped children and youth. Appl Res Ment Retard 1:55–69, 1980

23. Gualtieri CT, Guimond M: Tardive dyskinesia and the behavioral consequences of chronic neuroleptic treatment. Dev Med Child Neurol 23:255–259, 1981

24. Schroeder SR, Gualtieri CT: Behavioral interactions induced by chronic neuroleptic therapy in persons with mental retardation. Psychopharmacol Bull 21:310–315, 1985

25. Kane JM, Woerner M, Weinhold P, et al: A prospective study of tardive dyskinesia development: preliminary results. Clin Psychopharmacol 2:345–349, 1982

26. Glazer WM, Moore DC, Schooler, et al: Tardive dyskinesia: a discontinuation study. Arch Gen Psychiatry 41:623–627, 1984

27. Yassa R, Nair V, Schwartz G: Tardive dyskinesia: two-year follow-up study. Psychosomatics 25:852–855, 1984

28. Paulson GW, Rizvi CA, Crane GE: Tardive dyskinesia as a possible sequelae of long-term therapy with phenothiazines. Clin Pediatrics 14:953–955, 1975

29. Guy W: ECDEU Assessment Manual for Psychopharmacology. Washington, DC, Department Health, Education & Welfare, 1976

30. Gualtieri CT, Breuning SR, Sprague RL, et al: A centralized data system for studies of tardive dyskinesia in children, adolescents and the developmentally handicapped. Journal Supplement Abtract Service, Catalog of Selected Documents in Psychology, MS 2471, 1982

31. Jeste DV, Potkin SG, Sinha S, et al: Tardive dyskinesia—reversible and persistent. Arch Gen Psychiatry 36:585–590, 1979

32. Adams JH, Mitchell DE, Graham DK, et al: Diffuse brain damage of immediate impact type. Brain 100:489–502, 1977

33. Ommaya AK, Gennarelli TA: Cerebral concussion and traumatic unconsciousness: correlation of experimental and clinical observations on blunt head injuries. Brain 97:633–654, 1974

34. Itil TM, Soldatos C: Epileptogenic side effects of psychotropic drugs: practical recommendations. JAMA 244:1460–1463, 1980

35. Johnson FN: Psychoactive drugs and stimulus analysis: III. Adjustment of behavioral measures for drug-induced memory effects and state dependence: case of chlorpromazine. Int J Neurosci 20:25–32, 1983

36. Oliver AP, Luchins DJ, Wyatt RJ: Neuroleptic-induced seizures: an invitro technique for assessing relative risk. Arch Gen Psychiatry 39:206–209, 1984

37. Wise RA: Neuroleptics and operant behavior: the anhedonia hypothesis. Behav Brain Sci 5:39–87, 1982

38. Caine ED, Polinsky RJ: Haloperidol-induced dysphoria in patients with Tourette syndrome. Am J Psychiatry 136:1216–1217, 1979

39. Killan GA, Holzman PS, Davis JM, et al: Effects of psychotropic medication on selected cognitive and perceptual measures. J Abnorm Psychol 93:58–70, 1984

40. Kane JM, Smith JM: Tardive dyskinesia, prevalence and risk factors. Arch Gen Psychiatry 39:473–481, 1982

41. Wolf ME, Ryan J, Mosnaim AD: Cognitive functions in tardive dyskinesia. Psychol Med 13:671–674, 1983

42. Gardos G, Casey DE: Tardive Dyskinesia and Affective Disorders. Washington, DC, American Psychiatric Press, 1984

43. Wolf ME, DeWolfe AS, Ryan JJ, et al: Vulnerability to tardive dyskinesia. J. Clin Psychiatry 46:367–368, 1985

44. Divac I: Functions of the caudate nucleus. Acta Biol Exp 28:107–120, 1968

45. Buchwald NA, Hull CD, Levine MS, et al: The basal ganglia and the regulation of response and cognitive sets, in Growth and Development of the Brain. Edited by Brazier MAB. New York, Raven Press, 1975, pp. 171–189

46. Goldman PS, Alexander GE: Maturation of prefrontal cortex in the monkey revealed by local reversible cryogenic depression. Nature 267:613–615, 1977

Chapter 11

Tardive Dystonia: Diagnosis and Treatment

William C. Koller, M.D., Ph.D.

Chapter 11

Tardive Dystonia: Diagnosis and Treatment

Neuroleptic drugs are capable of inducing a variety of extrapyramidal syndromes including parkinsonism and hyperkinesias (1). Dyskinesias or hyperkinesias are characterized by a remarkable diversity of involuntary movements. Athetosis, particularly of the hands; chorea, often of the orofacial area; tics; myoclonus; and dystonia may be observed (2). This chapter reviews the dystonic syndromes, particularly tardive dystonia, that may result from neuroleptic therapy.

DYSTONIC SYNDROMES IN NEUROLOGICAL DISEASE

The term *dystonia* refers to the clinical manifestation of abnormal muscle contraction or spasms that result is involuntary, sustained twisting movements of body parts (3). The movements are relatively slow and sustained causing the maintenance of an abnormal posture. The nonpatterning, contorting movements can involve both axial and appendicular musculature and tend to be more proximal than distal. Their distribution may be generalized or segmental, affecting one body part. Dystonia may occur as a manifestation of diverse neurological conditions and can be induced by drugs.

When no discernible cause can be found in patients suffering from dystonia without other neurological impairments, these conditions are referred to as the primary dystonias (4, 5). Idiopathic torsion dystonia (dystonia musculorum deformans) is a disorder that may be inherited as an autosomal recessive trait in Ashkenazic Jews or an autosomal dominant trait in other ethnic groups, or may occur sporadically. The disease usually begins in childhood with inversion of the foot (foot dystonia). Intermittency of symptoms and exacerbation with stress are often encountered. Action dystonia, induction of the abnormal movement by a specific action, is common. The dystonia becomes generalized with the progression of the disease. No pathological substrate for torsion dystonia appears to exist. A variety of idiopathic dystonias are focal in nature involving selected muscles. Spasmodic torticollis is a focal dystonia that results from spasms of neck muscles causing the head to turn to one side (6). Retrocollis refers to the head turning backwards. Spasms of the muscles around the eyes (orbicularis oculi) result in a restricted dystonia called blepharospasm. The spasms may be so severe and frequent that functional blindness results. The combination of blepharospasm and dystonia of the oromandibular area is known by the eponym of Meige's syndrome (7). A spastic dysphonia results from a focal dystonia of the vocal cord muscles. Writer's cramp or the so-called occupational cramps or spasms are examples of focal dystonia affecting the hands (8).

There is very limited knowledge regarding the pathophysiology of dystonic disorders. Dystonia is thought to be due to basal ganglia dysfunction, particularly disturbances of the putamen (9). Disorders that primarily affect the basal ganglia may have dystonia as a part of their various clinical symptoms. These conditions can therefore be referred to as the symptomatic dystonias (10). Dystonia may be observed in patients with postencephalitic parkinsonism, Huntington's disease, Hallervoden-Spatz disease, or Wilson's disease. Besides these neurodegenerative disorders, other conditions that result in destructive lesions of the basal ganglia may cause dystonia. Cerebral palsy (perinatal injury), stroke, trauma, tumors, and infections can cause a dystonic disorder (11, 12). If the basal ganglia is affected unilaterally then a contralateral limb dystonia will result.

Drugs are also capable of inducing dystonia. Levodopa therapy of Parkinson's disease may cause dystonia in these patients. The anticonvulsants phenytoin and carbamazepine have been reported to cause dystonia in brain-damaged individuals (13, 14). Neuroleptic drugs can induce dystonia both as an acute and as a delayed or tardive syndrome.

ACUTE DYSTONIA

Acute dystonia occurs soon after treatment with neuroleptic drugs. These reactions may appear within hours of a single dose (1). It is estimated that 50 percent of cases occur within 48 hours of an initial dose and that 90 percent begin within 5 days of treatment. The incidence of acute dystonic reaction is thought to be 2 to 5 percent of patients who receive neuroleptics (15). Incidence rates tend to be higher in young adults, and men are more often affected than women. It appears that the more potent neuroleptic compounds, such as the butyrophenones and piperazine phenothiazines, are the primary drugs that induce acute dystonias. These compounds are also the most common drugs responsible for drug-induced parkinsonism.

Involvement of the muscles of the eyes, face, neck, and throat are common (15, 16). Oculogyric crisis and other averse eye movements, blepharospasm, trismus, forced jaw opening, grimacing, protrusion and twisting of the tongue, and distortion of the lips may be observed. Oculogyric crises usually result in upward conjugate deviation of the eyes. Patients may complain of eye pain or blurred or double vision. Spasmodic torticollis or retrocollis is common. Dystonia of the glossopharyngeal muscles may result in dysarthria, dysphagia, and respiratory stridor. The trunk tends to be more involved when children have the reaction. Opisthotonus, scoliosis, lordosis, trunk flexion, and tortipelvis may be observed. Limb dystonia can also occur. The clinical manifestations may fluctuate in severity and even in some cases spontaneously remit. A less pronounced form of dystonia with tightness of the jaw or difficulty with tongue movements may occur in some patients as an isolated phenomena or may precede a more severe dystonic reaction.

TARDIVE DYSTONIA

The ability of neuroleptic drugs to produce abnormal involuntary movement disorders with long-term treatment is well known. The predominant and characteristic movements are choreoathetotic, affecting the oral region, hands, and feet (tardive dyskinesia). Less commonly, other types of abnormal movements such as myoclonus, tics (Tourette-like syndrome), akathisia, or dystonia may be present (18–20). Occasionally dystonic movements will be the predominant late abnormal movements induced by neuroleptic drugs. Many reports document a dystonic syndrome with chronic therapy (21–44). The evidence of an etiological role of neuroleptic drugs in tardive dyskinesia is mainly epidemiological; however, the association is firmly established. Dystonia in psychiatric patients treated with neuroleptics is relatively rare, and the exact incidence of idiopathic dystonia in the general and psychiatric population is unknown. It is assumed that neuroleptic drugs can induce dystonic disorders with long-term treatment, but convincing epidemiological data are lacking at the current time. Criteria for diagnosing tardive dystonia include 1) the presence of chronic dystonia, 2) history of chronic neuroleptic exposure preceding or concurrent with the onset of dystonia, 3) exclusion of known causes of secondary dystonia by appropriate clinical and laboratory evaluation, and 4) a negative family history of dystonia. Dystonic symptoms as a late complication of neuroleptics have been reported to occur in 1 percent of 97 patients assessed for movement disorders by Crane and Naranjo (31) and 2 percent of 351 inpatients reported by Yassa et al. (32). Some of the patients labeled as tardive dystonia, could, of course, be examples of idiopathic torsion dystonia appearing coincidentally with neuroleptic drug use. Currently there is no way to distinguish idiopathic torsion dystonia from drug-induced dystonia.

The majority of cases reported have been young males. Gimenez-Rolden et al. compared 9 tardive dystonia cases to 13 patients with severe tardive dyskinesia (36). Both groups were neurological referrals from the same source. Advanced age and female preponderance were prominent features in the tardive dyskinesia group, while most of the tardive dystonia cases occurred in young adulthood with a slight majority of males. Age and female gender are thought to be important risk factors for the development of tardive dyskinesia (38). Neuroleptic compounds of different classes all appear capable of causing tardive dystonia (21–44). Similarly, specific neuroleptic drugs have not yet been shown to preferentially cause tardive dyskinesia (38). The duration of neuroleptic exposure has varied greatly in reported cases, and not enough information exists to define the length of treatment necessary to induce tardive dystonia. The average duration of exposure was 3.2 years in the cases of Burke et al. (29). There appears to be no correlation between the dose of neuroleptic and the emergence of tardive dystonia. Tardive dystonia is similar to tardive dyskinesia in that symptoms may abate following neuroleptic withdrawal. However, it is clear that patients suffer with dystonic movements for prolonged periods even after drug discontinuation. It appears that tardive dystonia has a fairly poor prognosis for reversibility. Significant recovery was found by Burke et al. (29) in only five of 42 patients. A much higher reversibility rate is thought to occur in tardive dyskinesia (45). However, while the remission rate in tardive dyskinesia following drug discontinuation has been somewhat defined (38), the small number of reported cases of tardive dystonia precludes similar types of analysis.

The clinical manifestations of the movements of tardive dystonia are diverse. Generalized dystonia, affecting all four limbs and the trunk, segmental dystonia, involving more than one body region, and focal dystonia, affecting a single body region, can occur. Opisthotonus, torticollis, retrocollis, focal limb dystonia, blepharospasm, oromandibular dystonia, combined blepharospasm-oromandibular dystonia (identical clinically to the idiopathic condition of Meige's syndrome), and marked axial dystonias have been described. Action dystonia, dystonic tremor, and pharyngeal dystonia have been observed with spasmodic dysphonia (42). Oculogyric crisis, common in acute dystonias, have been reported in several patients (39, 41). In general the dystonic movements begin insidiously, progress, and remain static therafter for a long period of time. It is not uncommon to have other types of abnormal movements present in addition to the dystonia. Choreatic movements typical of tardive dyskinesia are often present. Myoclonus, tics, and tremors may also be observed in combination with the dystonia (29). Marked functional disability may be associated with tardive dystonia. Opisthotonic and axial dystonias interface with gait, respiration, and speech. One patient was reported confined to a wheelchair because of action dystonia of the legs (37), and another patient was bedridden because of the dystonias (29). The dystonic movements appear to cause more problems for the patients than the choreatic movements of tardive dyskinesia. Certainly patients are much more aware of dystonic symptoms than choreatic movements and tend to complain about them.

The treatment of dystonic disorders is characterized by inconsistent and minimal responsiveness to most drugs (46). Recently the use of Botulinum A toxin has resulted in improvement of some idiopathic focal dystonias such as blepharospasm and torticollis (47). The therapy of tardive dystonia is usually unsatisfactory. A transient improvement of symptoms will occur in some patients when the dose of neuroleptics is increased (29). In the series of Burke et al. (29) some improvement was found in 68 percent of patient treated with tetrabenazine, a reserpine-like drug that depletes presynaptic dopamine, and in 39 percent of those receiving anticholinergic drugs. Wolf and Koller (37) studied three patients with prominent tardive dystonia and gave trihexiphenidyl, an anticholinergic, at doses of 20 mg/day. Improvement was minimal and transient, and moreover some preexisting choreatic movements were made worse by the therapy. Diazepam, propranolol, and clonazepam have been reported to be helpful to some patients (29). Several patients have been described who improved greatly with baclofen, 60 mg/day (32, 44). Bromocriptine, 40 mg/day, had marked benefit in one patient with torticollis thought to be due to chronic neuroleptic therapy (35). However, drug therapy in the majority of cases is unsuccessful, and for the most part tardive dystonia is refractory to treatment. Improvement of one patient with tardive dystonia who received electroconvulsive therapy for depression has been reported (33).

As with tardive dyskinesia (1), the early recognition of tardive dystonia and the withdrawal of neuroleptic drugs may result in remission and prevention of this condition.

REFERENCES

1. American Psychiatric Association, Task Force on Late Neurological Effects of Antipsychotic Drugs: Tardive Dyskinesia: Summary of a task force report of the American Psychiatric Association. Am J Psychiatry 137:1163–1173, 1980

2. Tarsy D, Baldessarini RJ: The tardive dyskinesia syndrome. Clin Neuropharmacol 1:29–61, 1976

3. Fahn S, Eldridge R: Definition of dystonia and classification of the dystonia. Adv Neurol 24:335–351, 1979

4. Eldridge R: The torsion dystonias: literature review and genetic and clinical studies. Neurology 20:1–78, 1970

5. Marsden CD, Harrison MJG: Idiopathic torsion dystonia: a review of 42 patients. Brain 97:793–810, 1974

6. Lal S, Hoyte K, Kiely ME: Neuropharmacological investigation and treatment of spasmodic torticollis. Adv Neurol 24:335–351, 1979

7. Toloso ES, Lai C: Meige syndrome striatal dopaminergic preponderance. Neurology 29:1126–1130, 1979

8. Sheehy MP, Marsden CD: Writer's cramp—a focal dystonia. Brain 105:461–480, 1982

9. Burton K, Fanrell K, Li D, et al: Lesions of the putamen and dystonia, CT and magnetic resonance imaging. Neurology 34:962–965, 1984

10. Zemar W, Whitlock CC: Symptomatic dystonias, in Handbook of Clinical Neurology (Volume 6). Edited by Vinkin PJ, Brayn GW. Amsterdam, Elsevier-North-Holland, 1968, pp.544–566

11. Maura AJ, Fahn S: Hemidystonia following "minor" head trauma. Trans Am Neurol Assoc 105:229–231, 1982

12. Demierre B, Rondot P: Dystonia caused by putamino-capsulo caudate vascular lesions. J Neurol Neurosurg 46:404–409, 1983

13. Chalub EG, DeVivo DC, Volpe JJ: Phenytoin-induced dystonia and choreoathetosis in two retarded epileptic children. Neurology 26:494–498, 1976

14. Crosley CJ, Swendee PT: Dystonia associated with carbamazepine administration experience in brain-damaged children. Pediatrics 63:612–615, 1979

15. Marsden CD, Tarsy D, Baldessarini RJ: Spontaneous and drug-induced movement disorders in psychiatric patients, in Psychiatric Aspects of Neurologic Disease. Edited by Benson DF, Blumer D. New York, Grune and Stratton, 1975, pp. 219–266

16. Klawans HC: Recognition and diagnosis of tardive dyskinesia. J Clin Psychiatry 46:3–7, 1985

17. Kolbe, A, Clon A, Jenner P, et al: Neuroleptic-induced acute dystonic reactions may be due to enhanced dopamine release or to supersensitive post-synaptic receptors. Neurology 31:434–439, 1981

18. Seeman MJ, Patel J, Pyhe J: Tardive dyskinesia with Tourette-like syndrome. J Clin Psychiatry 42:357–358, 1981

19. Weiner WJ, Ludy ED: Tardive akathesia. J Clin Psychiatry 44:417–419, 1983

20. Crane GE: Tardive dyskinesia in patients treated with major neuroleptics: a review of the literature. Am J Psychiatry 124:40–48, 1968

21. Dabbons IA, Bergman AB: Neurologic damage associated with phenothiazines. Am J Dis Child 111:291–296, 1966

22. Shields WB, Bray PF: A danger of haloperidol therapy in children. J Pediatr 88:301–303, 1976

23. Crane GE: Persistent dyskinesia. Br J Psychiatry 122:395–405, 1976

24. Druckman R, Seelinger D, Thulin B: Chronic involuntary movements induced by phenothiazines. J Nerv Ment Dis 135:69–76, 1962

25. Chaeau R, Fan R, Groslembert R, et al: A propos d'un cas de torticolis spasmodique irreversible surbenu au cors d'un traitement par neuroleptiques. Ann Med Psychol 122:1101–1111, 1966

26. Keegan DL, Rajput AH: Drug-induced dystonia tarda. Treatment with L-dopa. Dis Nerve Syst 38:167–169, 1973

27. Angle CR, McIntire MS: Persistent dystonia in a brain damaged child after ingestion of phenothiazine. J Pediatr 73:124–126, 1968

28. Harenko A: Retrocollis as an irreversible late manifestation of neuroleptic medication. Acta Neurol Scand 43:145–146, 1967

29. Burke RE, Fahn S, Jankovic J: Tardive dystonia: late onset and persistent dystonia caused by anti-psychotic drugs. Neurology 32:1335–1346, 1982

30. Degwitz R, Wenzel W: Persistent extrapyramidal side effects after long term application of neuroleptics, in Neuropsychology. Edited by Ball W. The Hague, Excerpta Medica, 1967, pp. 231–239

31. Crane GE, Naranjo ER: Motor disorders induced by neuroleptics: a proposed new classification. Arch Gen Psychiatry 24:179–184, 1971

32. Yassa R, Nair V, Dimitry R: Prevalence of tardive dystonia. Acta Psychiatr Scand 73:629–633, 1986

33. Kwenrus JA, Schalz C, Hart RP: Tardive dystonia, catatonia, an electroconvulsive therapy. J Nerv Ment Dis 132:171–173, 1984

34. Peatfield RC, Spokes ES: Phenothiazine-induced dystonias. Neurology 34:260, 1984

35. Lunchin DJ, Baldman M: High dose bromocriptine in a case of tardive dystonia. Biol Psychiatry 20:179–181, 1985

36. Gimenez-Roldan S, Mateo D, Bartolomi P: Tardive dyskinesia. Acta Psychiatr Scand 71:488–494, 1985

37. Wolf ME, Koller WC: Tardive dystonia treatment with trihexiphenidyl. J Clin Psychopharmacol 5:247–248, 1985

38. Kane JM, Smith JH: Tardive dyskinesia prevalence and risk factors: 1959 to 1979. Arch Gen Psychiatry 39:473–481, 1982

39. Nasrallah HA, Pappas NJ, Drane RR: Oculogyric dystonia in tardive dyskinesia. Am J Psychiatry 137:850–851, 1980

40. Gardos G: Dystonic reactions during maintenance antipsychotic therapy. Am J Psychiatry 138:114–115, 1981

41. Manetz MR: Oculogyric crisis and tardive dyskinesia. Am J Psychiatry 137:1628, 1980

42. Menuck M: Laryngeal–pharyngeal dystonia and haloperidol. Am J Psychiatry 138:394–395, 1981

43. Long AE: Dopamine agonists in the treatment of dystonia. Clin Neuropharmacol 8:38–57, 1985

44. Rosse RB, Allen A, Lux WE: Baclofen treatment in a patient with tardive dystonia. J Clin Psychiatry 47:474–475, 1986

45. Jeste DV, Potkin SG, Sinha S, et al: Tardive dyskinesia—reversible and persistent. Arch Gen Psychiatry 36:585–590, 1979

46. Fahn SP: Torsion dystonia: clinical spectrum and treatment. Semin Neurol 2:316–323, 1982

47. Jankovic J, Arman J: Botulinum A toxin for cranial–cervical dystonia: a double-blind placebo controlled study. Neurology 37:616–623, 1987

Chapter 12

Tardive Dyskinesia: Structural Changes in the Brain

K. R. Rama Krishnan, M.D.
Everett H. Ellinwood, Jr., M.D.
Krishnaiah Rayasam, M.D.

Chapter 12

Tardive Dyskinesia: Structural Changes in the Brain

Tardive dyskinesia (TD) is an extrapyramidal syndrome developing late in chronic treatment with neuroleptics. Clinical manifestations can vary from buccolinguo masticatory to choreathetoid movements, dystonia, and akathisia. Tardive dyskinesia may disappear in about 50 percent of patients after withdrawal of the neuroleptic (1), with a period that can vary up to 3 years; thus, the assessment of persistence and reversibility becomes problematic. The dyskinesia should be considered as persistent only after a period of 3, preferably drug-free, years (1). The underlying neuroanatomical substrate and pathophysiological basis of these varied movements (both reversible and irreversible) remains uncertain.

Since TD is more frequently observed in the elderly and is often irreversible, Crane (2) hypothesized the presence of predisposing organic factors and that the irreversibility reflected neuronal degeneration of the basal ganglia. Thus, one must bear in mind the distinction between predisposing organic factors and the putative damage by neuroleptics.

The most direct assessment of the neuroanatomical substrates are neuropathological studies, for which there are no reports of properly controlled studies. Hunter et al. (3) in an open study of three cases of TD found that in only one subject were there significant findings, for example, black staining material in the globus pallidus, pallidofuigal fibres, and capsule of the subthalamic nucleus and in the upper part of the substantia nigra to reflect Wallerian degeneration. Christensen et al. (4) studied 28 patients with dyskinesias, 21 of whom had TD, and 28 controls matched by diagnosis. They found that cell

This work was supported in part by a Clinical Associate Physician Supplement to RR-30 General Clinical Research Center Program, National Institutes of Health.

degeneration in the substantia nigra and gliosis in the midbrain and brainstem were more frequent in subjects with dyskinesia. Ventricular dilatation and cortical atrophy were also more frequently seen in dyskinetic patients. This study suffered from 1) poor matching of controls on age, sex, and duration of neuroleptic therapy; 2) nonblind assessment of case material; and 3) inclusion of a mixed group of dyskinetic patients. Besides these two studies, there is a case report by Campbell et al. (5) of increased iron deposition in the basal ganglia and substantia nigra in a patient with TD.

Postmortem studies of patients with TD have been limited so far and the results difficult to generalize. The other studies that have assessed neuroanatomical changes have been done primarily with computerized axial tomography and more recently with magnetic resonance imaging.

COMPUTERIZED TOMOGRAPHY IN PATIENTS WITH TARDIVE DYSKINESIA

Gelenberg (6) studied eight chronic schizophrenic patients with TD between the ages of 17 and 56; the dyskinesia had persisted for at least 4 months. He used three computerized tomography (CT) cuts per subject, and the results were interpreted in a qualitative rather than a quantitative manner. One subject had mild generalized cortical atrophy, and none of the subjects were reported as having significantly abnormal scans.

Jeste et al. (7) studied 12 elderly female patients with TD and 12 control subjects, matched for age, sex, primary psychiatric diagnosis, and length of neuroleptic treatment. Ten patients in each group suffered from schizophrenia, and the remaining two pairs of subjects had organic brain syndrome. The duration of TD was not given although it was noted that symptoms ranged in duration from months to years. Five TD patients were noted to be drug free for months. An average of 12 CT cuts were obtained per subject, and quantitative analysis was done using 1) bifrontal bicaudate ratio (8), Hahn's cerebroventricular indices (9), ventricular brain ratio (VBR) (10), Huckman's criteria for cortical atrophy (11), and Allen's criteria for cerebellar atrophy (12). Jeste et al. (7) noted no differences between patients with and without TD on any of these measures.

Famuyiwa et al. (13) studied 17 schizophrenic patients with TD and 33 patients without TD. All patients were below the age of 60, and they did not significantly differ from each other on the basis of age, sex, duration of hospitalization, duration of treatment, or social class. The duration of TD and its persistence after drug withdrawal was not mentioned in the report. The scanning procedure was not described. Ventricular enlargement and cerebral atrophy were graded qualitatively on a 0-to-3-point scale. Huckman's number (11), ventricular index (14) and cell media index (14) were also measured. The two groups were reported to differ only on ventricular index. More patients with TD had an abnormal ventricular index than patients without TD. Since the cutoff point used for assessing an abnormal ventricular index was arbitrary and based on a prior study and the validity of such a measure was not discussed, the significance of this observation remains open to question.

Jeste et al. (15) in a study of six male schizophrenic patients below the age of 50 with TD and six matched controls (7) confirmed the already reported lack of difference between the two groups (7).

Brainin et al. (16) studied 15 patients (age range = 20 to 59 years) with TD. The duration of this condition was not mentioned, and no control group was included; instead, values were compared to those of a normal population. Each subject had eight cuts on CT examination, and the measures used were the ventricle index ratio, ventricular waist ratio, and a qualitative assessment of cortical atrophy. Although four patients showed some signs of atrophy, they found no difference between patients with TD and the normal population.

Owens et al. (17) investigated lateral ventricular size in 112 institutionalized chronic schizophrenic patients. CT scan procedure was not described. Lateral ventricular size was assessed by using the VBR (10), and a relationship between VBR and severity of abnormal movements, as measured by the Abnormal Involuntary Movements Scale (AIMS), was reported. However, no mention was made about the nature, duration, and persistence of the abnormal movements. This study did not specifically address the issue of neuroanatomical change in patients with TD and therefore did not use a matched control sample.

Kaufmann et al. (18) studied VBR of 32 patients with TD and 57 controls; the groups were not matched. The patients included those previously reported by Jeste et al. (7, 15). The CT scanning procedure was not described. Patients with TD had a trend toward larger VBRs than those without TD, but difference in VBR between the two groups was lost when age was used as a covariable. There was also no difference in bifrontal/bicaudate ratio between patients with TD (n = 30) and without TD (n = 53).

Albus et al. (19) studied 24 schizophrenic patients with TD and 15 controls matched to diagnosis. There was no difference between the two groups in terms of age, age of onset of illness, or duration of neuroleptic treatment. Duration and persistence of TD was not given. CT scans were obtained with 12 cuts per subject. The following were measured: VBR (10), Huckman's criteria for cortical atrophy (11), width of third ventricle, maximal width of anterior horns of lateral ventricle, and distance between both choroid plexuses. They found that patients with severe TD had wider sulci as measured by the Huckman criteria than patients without TD.

Kolakowska et al. (20), using CT, studied 12 schizophrenic patients with TD and 26 patients without TD. The groups were not matched. However, there was no difference between the groups in terms of age and years since first neuroleptic treatment. The duration and persistence of TD were not mentioned and CT scanning procedure was not described. Although only VBR was measured, the VBR data were not presented; instead the number of subjects who had large ventricles (>1 SD on the VBR) was given. There was no difference between the two groups on this measure.

The design, methodology, and results of these studies are summarized in Table 1. It is clear that the methodology varied considerably. Further, the measurement techniques also varied and no index of reliability was given in any study. Patient population varied and none of the studies assessed mentioned duration and persistence of TD. The matching of controls to TD patients also varied across studies. Despite these shortcomings there was little evidence of neuroanatomical changes relating particularly to TD. One reason may be that CT is not sensitive enough to detect neuroanatomical changes of relevance to TD, that is, ability to detect changes in the basal ganglia. Evidence for this comes from studies of Huntington's chorea where CT scan changes were seen only in some subjects (21). An important problem with CT studies is that the neuroanatomical changes seen are not specific; for example, ventricular dilation, cerebral atrophy, etc. are also present in a wide range of conditions, such as schizophrenia, bipolar disorder, and Alzheimer's disease. Thus, even if some of these changes are seen in CT studies of TD patients, it will be impossible to relate them directly to TD patients, but can only point to TD, especially when the changes are seen in TD patients with primary conditions not known to be related to CT scan abnormalities. The advent of magnetic resonance imaging (MRI) seems to provide a more sensitive method for assessing neuroanatomical changes in this condition.

MRI IN TARDIVE DYSKINESIA

Nuclear magnetic resonance has evolved from a method of measuring the magnetic properties of atoms to a tool which is used to study the structure and concentration of molecules in biological tissues.

Table 1. Summary of Computerized Tomography Studies in Patients with Tardive Dyskinesia (TD)

Study	TD n	Controls n	Cortical atrophy Measure used	Cortical atrophy Yes/No	Ventricular dilatation Measure used	Ventricular dilatation Yes/No	Cerebellar changes (Yes/No)	Third ventricle enlargement (Yes/No)	Caudate atrophy
Brainin et al. (16)	15	Normals	Qualitative	No	VIR/VWR	No	Not done	Not done	Not done
Famuyiwa et al. (13)	17	33	Huckman	No	VIR	Yes	Not done	No	Not done
Gelenberg (6)	8	None	Qualitative	1 had mild change	Qualitative	No	Not done	Not done	Not done
Jeste et al. (7)	12	12	Huckman	No	VBR	No	No*	Not done	BF–BC normal
Jeste et al. (15)	6	6	Huckman	No	VBR	No	No*	Not done	BF–BC normal
Kaufman et al. (18)	32	57	Huckman	No	VBR	No	No*	Not done	Not done
Owens et al. (17)	Total of 112 points not designated as TD or non-TD.		Not done	—	VBR	Yes	Not done	Not done	Not done
Albus et al. (19)	21	15	Width of 4 largest sulci	Yes	VBR	No	Not done	None	Not done
Kolakowska et al. (20)	12	26	Not done	—	VBR	No	Not done	Not done	Not done

Note. Yes/No refers to the presence or absence of significant difference between patients and controls. VIR = ventricular index ratio; VWR = ventricular waist ratio; VBR = ventricular brain ratio; BF–BC = bifrontal bicaudate ratio.
*All these studies used Allen's criteria for cerebeller changes.

The advantages of MRI are related to the fact that the images are synthesized from a multitude of parameters, a number far larger than any other imaging modality, and provide tomographic images with excellent spatial and anatomical resolution. MRI in humans today consists primarily of data acquired about hydrogen density (the most prevalent atom in humans), and the scans provide information through measurement of T_1 and T_2 relaxation times of the physicochemical environment surrounding the hydrogen proton. With MRI a multitude of techniques yielding a spectrum of information can be used to provide images, for example, spin echo, inversion recovery, and saturation recovery. Further, by altering different parameters in these sequences, such as pulse interval or spin echo delay time, and by varying the thickness of the slices, the gaps between slices, the directions and planes of imaging, a great variety of images can be generated. This ability is a tremendous advantage of MRI (22).

Of particular relevance to TD is that MRI permits an excellent resolution of basal ganglia structures. Further, aside from producing superb neuroanatomical structures it may also provide unique biochemical information about brain function. A decrease in signal intensity on spin echo sequence with relaxation time of 2000 ms and echo delay time of 100 ms reflects an increase in ferric iron. The decrease in T_2 measurement in basal ganglia stress correlates with increased ferric iron in these structures (23). Brain iron is present in the form of ferritin and as a cofactor of important enzymes, including tyrosine hydroxylase, tryptophan hydroxylase, and aldehyde oxidase. Iron is also believed to be involved in dopamine function (24). Iron concentrations in the basal ganglia are increased in various degenerative disorders including Hallevorden Spatz disease, Huntington's disease, and Parkinson's disease (25). Thus, changes in iron may prove to be a more specific marker of neuronal degeneration in the basal ganglia of patients with TD. Since a recent neuropathological study in TD (5) noted increased iron pigment in the basal ganglia, it is possible that degeneration of the neurons of the basal ganglia in TD may be reflected in increased iron concentration in these structures. Studies to assess this change in iron are currently underway.

At present there is only one published study of MRI in TD (26). Besson et al. (25) studied 21 patients with schizophrenia, 6 of whom had TD. There was no difference between patients and controls in terms of structural changes but patients with TD had higher T_1 values in the basal ganglia than controls. The significance of this increase in T_1 is not known. T_1 is altered by a variety of factors, the major ones being changes in the water content and the ratio between free and bound water.

We have recently studied seven schizophrenic patients with MRI to assess changes in iron concentration in the basal ganglia. In this preliminary study we found that significant changes in iron concentration were not seen in these patients. But as in CT studies of schizophrenic patients, we found a significant increase in abnormalities such as cerebral atrophy, ventricular dilation, and leucodystrophy.

In summary, neuropathological, CT, and MRI studies reveal neuroanatomical and physicochemical changes in the brain of TD patients, but the exact nature and significance of these changes remain an enigma. We have reviewed the literature and attempted to assess the sources of variance, which include the patient population, the control groups used, the type and severity of TD, the question of "persistent TD," the methods of assessing neuroanatomical changes, and the measurement methods (that is, qualitative versus quantitative, different types of quantitative measures, and so forth). We shall briefly assess the potential impact of these sources of variance.

SOURCES OF VARIANCE

Patient Population

Patient populations in the studies generally consisted of patients with schizophrenia and organic brain syndrome. However, the age and duration of illness and the type of patients in terms of chronic institutionalized versus outpatients vary across studies. These sources of variance are particularly important, since neuropathological abnormalities similar to those reported in TD are frequently seen in patients with schizophrenia, especially patients with negative-symptom schizophrenia (27). Studying schizophrenic patients with TD will obscure the identification of possible neuroanatomical changes in TD. Further, since changes seen in patients with this condition are similar to what is reported in aging and institutionalized patients, studying primarily older patients with TD will also obscure the results of neuroanatomical studies.

Control Groups

The control groups used varied. Some studies had no control groups, others used normal subjects. Few controlled for duration of neuroleptic treatment, diagnosis, and age; since all of these variables may themselves account for the neuroanatomical changes observed, failure to control for these variables obscures the significance of the result reported.

Type and Severity of TD

While the typical buccofaciolingual syndrome is the most common type of TD, dystonic movements and akathisia may also be seen. To assume, as most of the uncontrolled studies do, that the pathophysiology underlying all types of TD and all grades of severity is the same is naive.

"Persistent" TD

Tardive dyskinesia refers to abnormal involuntary movements that start usually at least 6 months or more after the beginning of neuroleptic treatment. In up to 50 percent of patients these movements disappear after discontinuation of the medication. It is possible that the form of TD where these movements disappear may be caused by a mechanism different from the form of TD that does not disappear (persistent TD). Supersensitivity of D-2 receptors may be responsible for reversible TD, but it is possible that persistent TD may be caused by other receptor changes and by neuronal degeneration. None of the neuroanatomical studies specifically addressed this question.

Methods of Assessing Neuroanatomical Changes

The methods have varied from neuropathological studies to CT and MRI studies. Even within CT studies the type and number of cuts have varied, making it difficult to compare studies.

Measurement Methods

The methods of measurement have varied even across CT studies; some studies used qualitative and others used quantitative assessments. Even the type of quantitative assessments used and the types of neuroanatomical changes measured differed across studies; for example, some studied only the size of ventricles, others only cortical atrophy, making it difficult to compare studies.

As can be seen from this review, conceiving and conducting a well-designed study of neuroanatomical changes in TD is difficult. The results so far are inconclusive. The ideal approach would be a prospective postmortem neuropathological study of patients with TD with matched controls. Such a study however, would be very difficult to conduct. Neuroradiological studies must also be conducted in a prospective manner. To assess the issue of whether organic changes predispose toward the development of TD, it would be important to follow a group of schizophrenic patients with and without organic changes as assessed by MRI prospectively. To assess whether neuroleptics lead to neuronal changes in patients who develop TD, it would be important to assess neuroanatomical changes (preferably in a serial fashion with MRI) in patients with TD who are unlikely to exhibit neuroanatomical changes secondary to their primary condition. Further, such studies should address the question of identifying and studying more specific markers of neuronal degeneration in basal ganglia such as iron changes. Since the incidence of TD is more often increased in the elderly and neuroanatomical changes such as cerebral atrophy, ventricular dilation and leukodystrophy are more commonly seen in this population, the interaction between these variables, the dose of neuroleptics, the duration of exposure to neuroleptic in relation to the development and persistence of TD must be undertaken to more definitively answer the question whether these factors predispose toward the development of this condition.

REFERENCES

1. MacKay AVP: Clinical controversies in tardive dyskinesia, in Movement Disorders. Edited by Marsden CD, Fahn S. Butterworth, London, 1981.

2. Crane GE: Persistent dyskinesia. Br J Psychiatry 122:395–405, 1973

3. Hunter R, Blackwood W, Smith MC, et al: Neuropathological findings in three cases of persistent dyskinesia following phenothiazene medication. J Neurol Sci 7:268–273, 1978

4. Christensen E, Moller J, Faurbye A: Neuropathological investigation of 28 brains from patients with dyskinesia. Acta Psychiatr Scand 46:14–23, 1970

5. Campbell WG, Raskind MA, Gordon T, et al: Iron pigment in the brain of a man with tardive dyskinesia. Am J Psychiatry 142:364–365, 1985

6. Gelenberg AJ: Computerized tomography in patients with tardive dyskinesia; Am J Psychiatry 133:578–579, 1976

7. Jeste DV, Wagner RL, Weinberger DR, et al: Evaluation of CT scans in tardive dyskinesia. Am J Psychiatry 137:247–248, 1980

8. Neophytides AN, Dichiro G, Barron SA, et al: Computed axial tomography in Huntington's disease and persons at risk for Huntington's disease, in Advances in Neurology (Volume 23). Edited by Chase TN, Wesler NS, Barbeau A. New York, Raven Press, 1979, pp. 185–191

9. Hahn FJY, Rim K, Schapiro RL: A quantitative analysis of ventricular size on computerized tomography scans. Computed Tomography 1:121–125, 1977

10. Weinberger DR, Torrey EF, Neophytides AN, et al: Lateral cerebral ventricular enlargement in chronic schizophrenia. Arch Gen Psychiatry 36:735–739, 1979

11. Huckman MS, Fox J, Topel J: The validity of criteria for evaluation of cerebral atrophy by computed tomography. Radiology 116:85–92, 1975

12. Allen JH, Martin JT, McLain LW: Computerized tomography in cerebellar atrophic process. Radiology 130:379–381, 1978

13. Famuyiwa OO, Eccleston D, Donaldson AA, et al: Tardive dyskinesia and dementia. Br J Psychiatry 135:500–504, 1979

14. Meese W, Lanksch W, Wende S: Cerebral atrophy and computerized tomography, in Cranial Computerized Tomography. Edited by Lanksch W, Kazner E. New York, Springer Verlag, 1976, p. 22

15. Jeste DV, Weinberger DR, Zalcman S, et al: Computered tomography in tardive dyskinesia. Br J Psychiatry 136:606–608, 1980

16. Brainin M, Reisner IT, Zeitlhofer J: Tardive dyskinesia: clinic correlation with computed tomography in patients aged less than 60 years. J Neurol Neurosurg Psychiatry 46:1037–1040, 1983

17. Owens DGC, Johnstone EC, Crow TJ, et al: Lateral ventricular size in schizophrenia: relationship to the disease process and its clinical manifestations. Psychol Med 15:27–41, 1985

18. Kaufmann CA, Jeste DV, Shelton RC, et al: Nonadrenergic and neuroradiological abnormalities in tardive dyskinesia. Biol Psychiatry 21:799–812, 1986

19. Albus M, Naber D, Muller-Spahn E, et al: Tardive dyskinesia: relation to computer tomographic, endocrine, and psychopathological variables. Biol Psychiatry 20:1082–1089, 1985

20. Kolakowska T, Williams AO, Ardern M, et al: Tardive dyskinesia in schizophrenics under 60 years of age. Biol Psychiatry 21:161–169, 1986

21. Oepen G, Ostertag CH: Diagnostic values of CT in patients with Huntington's disease and their offspring. J Neurol 225:189–196, 1981

22. Margulis AR, Higgins CB, Kaufman L, et al: Clinical Magnetic Resonance Imaging. San Francisco, Radiology Research Education Foundation, 1985

23. Drayer BP, Burger P, Darwin R, et al: MRI of brain iron. Am J Radiology 147:103–110, 1986

24. Youdim MBH, Yehuda S, Ben-Shachar D, et al: Behavioral and brain biochemical changes in iron deficient rates: the involvement of iron and dopamine receptor function, in Iron Deficiency Brain Biochemistry and Behavior. Edited by Pollitt E, Leibel RL. New York, Raven Press, 1982, pp. 39–56

25. Park BE, Netsky MG, Betsill WL: Pathogenesis of pigment and spherocid formation in Hallevorden Spatz syndrome and related disorders. Neurology 25:1172–1178, 1975

26. Besson JAO, Corrigan FM, Cherryman GR, et al: Nuclear magnetic resonance brain imaging in chronic schizophrenia. Br J Psychiatry 150:161–163, 1987

27. Goetz KL, Van Kammen DP: Computerized axial tomography scans and subtypes of schizophrenia. J Nerv Ment Dis 174:31–41, 1986

Chapter 13

Neuroendocrine Aspects of Tardive Dyskinesia: The Role of Estrogen, Prolactin, and Dopamine

William M. Glazer, M.D.
Henry A. Nasrallah, M.D.

Chapter 13

Neuroendocrine Aspects of Tardive Dyskinesia: The Role of Estrogen, Prolactin, and Dopamine

Tardive dyskinesia (TD) is a movement disorder thought to be due to supersensitivity of nigrostriatal dopamine (DA) receptors induced by the chronic administration of antipsychotic medications (1). This hypothesis remains unproved despite numerous pharmacological studies. Clearly, it is important to consider other possible mechanisms that may contribute to this disorder. Over the last 10 years, there has been a rapidly growing interest in the effect of hormones, particularly gonadal hormones on central nervous system function (2). Gonadal hormones affect both the structure and function of brain areas during various stages of human development. In this chapter, we review basic and clinical data that point to the possibility that estrogen (EST) and prolactin (PRL) impact on the central nervous system at the time of menopause to contribute to the pathophysiology of TD.

It is unclear why only certain patients develop TD. One of the few risk factors that has been solidly implicated in the epidemiology of TD is increasing age (3, 4). Older female patients have been reported in several retrospective studies to be at greater risk for TD (5–7). Antipsychotic or neuroleptic drugs stimulate PRL secretion via DA receptor blocking effects on the tuberoinfundibular system (8–10).

Some patients demonstrate persistent elevation of serum PRL during chronic antipsychotic drug treatment. Since long-term administration of antipsychotic medication is associated with TD and elevated PRL levels, Glazer et al. (11) examined the relationship between PRL and TD in a population of neuroleptic-treated outpatients.

Glazer et al.'s study included 19 males and 29 postmenopausal females from the Yale Tardive Dyskinesia Clinic (12, 13). These patients with research diagnoses of TD were compared to 21 neuroleptic-treated men free of involuntary movements. Blood was obtained from patients at a standard time following a 12-hour fast, and serum PRL was assayed with a double-antibody radioimmunoassay.

Although there was no difference in PRL levels between the TD and non-TD males, the mean PRL level in the female TD group (29.1 ± 32.7 ng/ml) was significantly (p < .05) higher than that of the male TD group (12.0 ± 7.2 ng/ml). This finding replicated the earlier observation that women have higher PRL values than men after exposure to neuroleptic medication (14). When patients were divided according to sex and severity of TD, that is, mild (score of less than 6 on the Abnormal Involuntary Movement Scale [AIMS]) and severe (AIMS score higher than 6), it was found that the 14 women with severe TD had a significantly (p < .05) higher mean serum PRL (41.8 ± 41.7 ng/ml) compared to the 15 women with mild TD (18.3 ± 14.3 ng/ml). Such a difference was not evident in the male group. Further univariate analyses revealed no statistically significant association between PRL or TD severity and neuroleptic dose, use of other medication, and psychiatric diagnosis.

The results of this study raised two themes relevant to the neuroendocrinology of TD:

1. There is a sex-related association between PRL levels and severity of TD. The loss of EST in the postmenopausal group could impact on nigrostriatal DA function to account for this association.
2. Prolactin itself could play a role in the pathogenesis of TD through an interaction with the nigrostriatal DA system.

We shall discuss each theme separately.

ESTROGEN, STRIATAL DOPAMINE, AND TD

EST has been the subject of scientific investigation since the beginning of the 20th century and is known to exert various effects on the central nervous system function (15). Specific cytoplasmic and nuclear binding sites for estradiol have been identified biochemically (9, 10) and anatomically in the central nervous system (16–18). Kelly et al. (19) used electrophysiological techniques to demonstrate that 17-beta-estradiol succinate exerts an effect on the central nervous system. It is not yet clear whether EST can function by itself as a neuromodulator, but there is accumulating evidence that it interacts with cathecholamine systems in the brain. Mueller (20) and McEwen et al. (15) review biochemical evidence for EST effect on cathecholamine metabolism, release, and uptake.

Recently, several groups of investigators have become interested in studying EST–DA interactions at the nigrostriatal level. This interest has been stimulated in part by the clinical observation of movement disorders such as TD occurring in postmenopausal women (21, 22), chorea of pregnancy (23) and chorea induced by oral contraceptives (24). The study of the effect of EST on striatal DA in animals has occurred from behavioral, biochemical, and electrophysiological perspectives. A review of this literature is beyond the scope of this chapter, and the reader is referred to the work of Hruska (25). Selected electrophysiological studies are summarized in Table 1. In short, the animal literature strongly suggests that EST exerts an influence on striatal DA systems. The data are still confusing as to the precise mechanism(s) of action underlying this influence, so that a case may be made for EST's having either a positive or a negative effect on striatal DA function. Reasons for these conflicting reports include sex and species studied, housing conditions, type of EST used, as well as dose, route, and timing of administration (26).

Another explanation for these conflicting reports is that the effect of EST on striatal DA systems is modulatory in nature. Chiodo (26) suggests that EST has a complex modulatory rather than a neurotransmitter action on striatal DA in that it alters DA's dynamic range of responsiveness and thus potentiates the effect of pharmacological and environmental influences that both increase and decrease DA activity.

Menopause as a risk factor in TD (5, 32) is consistent with the idea of a modulatory influence of EST since it is also well known that estradiol levels fall during menopause. To develop this line of reasoning, Glazer et al. (33) measured serum EST levels in 43 of the 48 patients from the PRL study mentioned above. All of these neuroleptic-treated patients met research criteria for TD, and 25 (58.1 percent) were postmenopausal women. EST and PRL were measured by specific radioimmunoassay, and homovanillic acid (HVA) was measured by gas chromatography–mass spectroscopy using deuterated internal standards. As predicted, the women had a significantly (p < .005) lower estradiol level (mean = 19.8, SD = ±10.1 pg/ml) compared to the men (mean = 29.8, SD = ±12.0 pg/ml).

Estradiol levels did not correlate significantly with TD severity in the postmenopausal females. This finding was not too surprising since the population studied was limited to hypogonadal women. While a hypogonadal state could be a factor influencing the severity of TD, the data from this study suggest that the degree of hypo-

Table 1. Electrophysiological studies of estrogen's influence on striatal dopamine.

Reference	Animal studied	Method	Results
Bueno and Pfaff (27)	Ovariectomized female rats	Single unit recording in undefined heterogeneous populations of neurons located in the hypothalamus and preoptic areas. Estrogen (EST) was administered systemically intravenously.	EST tended to depress the spontaneous activity of preoptic cells and increase the number of cells firing in the hypothalamus.
Kelly et al. (19)	Adult female rats	Microiontophoresis of 17-Beta-estradiol hemisuccinate onto septal preoptic neurons.	Measured a direct inhibitory action of 17-Beta-estradiol hemisuccinate on septal preoptic neurons. Also demonstrated inhibitory and excitatory properties of 17-Beta-estradiol hemisuccinate (depending on the time of estrous cycle) in non-antidromically identified medial preoptic septal neurons.
Chiodo and Caggiula (28)	Ovariectomized female rats	Isolate single dopamine neurons within the zona compacta of the substantia nigra. 17-Beta-estradiol (10 µg/kg subcutaneously) given 2 and 10 days prior to recording. They then challenged with intravenous apomorphine (2 or 4 µg/kg).	We believe data pertaining to the B cells are most relevant. EST treatment 2 days but *not* 10 days prior to recording attenuated the ability of apomorphine to inhibit discharge of B cells.

Table 1. (continued)

Reference	Animal studied	Method	Results
		Examine effect of 17-Beta-estradiol (3, 30, 300, 3000 ng/kg intravenously) on the spontaneous firing of dopamine cells.	Measured a dose-dependent decrease in the activity of B cells.
Arnauld et al. (29)	Ovariectomized female rats; one group hypophysectomized	Estrogen benzoate 20 μg in sesame oil intramuscularly. Record unit activities from the caudate.	Estradiol reversed the dopamine sensitivity of caudate neurons.
		The electrical activity of caudate neurons and their response to iontophoretically applied dopamine were tested at different time intervals before and after intramuscular injections of estradiol benzoate.	EST reversed the sensitivity of caudate neurons to dopamine. These results were abolished by hypophysectomy.
Chiodo and Caggiula (30)	Ovariectomized female rats	Acute study of effect of 17-Beta-estradiol (intravenous) in 3, 30, 300, and 3000 ng/kg on spontaneous activity of Type A and B cells in zona compacta.	Increased Type A and decreased Type B cells in dose-dependent manner. Suggests that EST effect is on membrane, not cytosolic receptors.

Table 1. (continued)

Reference	Animal studied	Method	Results
		Sensitivity of autoreceptors examined (48 hours after subcutaneous 17-Beta-estradiol 10µg/kg) by measuring extent to which intravenous apomorphine (2 and 4 µg/kg) and microinotophoretically applied dopamine depressed spontaneous neuronal discharge.	EST treatment increased the response of Type A neurons and decreased that of Type B to apomorphine and dopamine.
Chiodo et al. (31)	Male rats	Examine effect of 17-Alpha- and Beta-estradiol on spontaneous activity of substantia nigral dopamine cell activity.	Beta-estradiol inhibited dopamine neurons firing starting at 1.2 µg/kg and all cells were inhibited at 19.2 µg/kg.
		Examine effect of 17-Beta-estradiol (0.6 or 1.2 µg/kg intravenously) 1–3 minutes before beginning sequential administration of apomorphine.	No effect of acute intravenous administration of EST on apomorphine dose–response curve.
		Examine effect of 10% 17-Beta-estradiol sialastic capsule implant for 2–3 hours prior to systematic administration of apomorphine. Cells-per-track method used in substantia area.	EST significantly reduced the number of spontaneously active dopamine neurons found.

gonadism is not important. Interestingly, when stepwise multiple regression analysis was performed with the AIMS score as the outcome variable, and PRL, estradiol HVA, and age as predictors, sex differences were observed. In the male group, there were no significant predictors of AIMS score. In the female group, HVA was the only significant predictor of TD severity, accounting for 14 percent of the variance (p = .06). While one must interpret cautiously the degree to which plasma HVA validly reflects central DA function, these results suggest a relationship between TD and DA function in postmenopausal women but not in men. Since the women in this sample had significantly lower estradiol levels compared to the men, it is possible that the loss of EST facilitates a sex-specific association between HVA and TD. A case control study of estradiol levels that controls for menopause, TD, and neuroleptic exposure would be an important future study.

These findings are consistent with the Bedard et al. (21) hypothesis that EST serves a protective role against neuroleptic-induced striatal DA pathology. Villeneuve et al. (22) conducted an open-label and double-blind study of EST therapy in TD and demonstrated a value in the use of conjugated estrogens for TD in a male population. Studies of the effect of EST on animal models of TD have been conducted. The administration of estradiol benzoate (8 µg/kg) to ovariectomized rats withdrawn from chronic haloperidol treatment prevented the usual increase in striatal dopamine receptor sites and apomorphine-induced stereotypy associated with this withdrawal (34, 35). Bedard et. al. (36) studied the effect of estradiol on a persistent oral dyskinesia produced by a midbrain lesion in four ovariectomized monkeys. The investigators reported that estradiol, given either chronically (several days) or acutely, antagonized the apomorphine-induced potentiation of the dyskinesia. They also reported a biphasic effect of the single (acute) 0.5 mg injection of estradiol on the movement disorder. At 24 hours after the injection, there was an inhibition of apomorphine, while at 3 days to 2 weeks there was a facilitation. These animal studies along with Villeneuve's work with a male TD population provided a basis for the following study.

Glazer et al. (37) examined EST replacement as a treatment for TD in postmenopausal women. This study employed a random assignment, double-blind, placebo-controlled design to test the efficacy of 3 weeks of conjugated estrogen (Premarin 1.25 mg/day) replacement therapy. Ten women included for study met research criteria for TD, had not had a menstrual period for at least a year, and had one or more signs and symptoms of estrogen deficiency. All patients received their usual neuroleptic maintenance therapy over the 3-week study period. Four exams, one at baseline, and the remaining three on a once-weekly basis, focused on TD movements, parkinsonian signs, and psychological symptoms. During the 3-week treatment period, all patients in the EST treatment group improved. The mean AIMS score decreased by 38 percent (range = 17 to 50 percent) in the EST group and by 9 percent in the placebo group. Figure 1 displays the mean AIMS and Webster (parkinsonism) scores for the treatment and placebo groups at the four time points studied. Although the difference in mean improvement was not statistically significant at the second and third exams, the difference was marginally significant at visit 4 (p = 0.09). Using repeated measures modeling, a greater average rate of improvement was seen in the EST-treated group compared to the placebo-treated group (p = .10). There were no significant differences between treatment groups for parkinsonian signs or psychological symptoms.

The results of this study suggest that EST replacement therapy is beneficial for TD in some postmenopausal women. The efficacy of

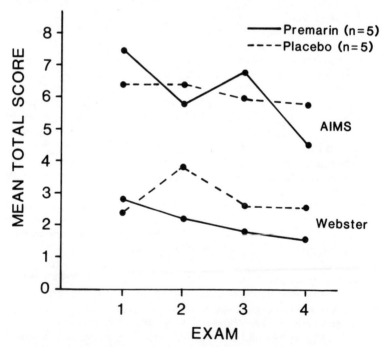

Figure 1.   Mean AIMS and Webster Scores in postmenopausal women receiving Premarin or placebo.

EST treatment further supports the idea that estrogen protects the nigrostriatal DA system from neuroleptic-induced pathology. This treatment strategy requires a collaboration between a psychiatrist and a gynecologist who can monitor patient selection and response on an ongoing basis. Efficacy of EST therapy can be established after about 3 weeks of treatment. It is important to keep in mind that the long-term value of EST replacement therapy for TD is not yet clear. In view of the findings from animal studies, it is possible that the efficacy of EST therapy may be seen only acutely. Given the concern raised about endometrial cancer from chronic EST exposure in the last 10 years (38), the chronic use of EST should be considered in risk–benefit terms. However, recently there has been a reconsideration of the risk-benefit ratio of EST replacement therapy (39).

The following is a case report suggesting that EST may be effective in ameliorating TD symptoms where several other approaches have failed.

Case Report

A 69-year-old white single female was referred for management of severe abnormal involuntary movements of 15 years duration. The patient had had several episodes of paranoid psychosis starting at age 43 years, for which she received neuroleptic treatment for approximately 22 years. Abnormal movements were first observed at age 44, after 1 year of neuroleptic therapy, and became progressively worse, especially after total discontinuation of neuroleptics 5 years prior to referral. She had no recurrence of psychotic symptoms after the discontinuation of neuroleptics, but had become almost disabled because of her continuous and severe involuntary movements of her tongue, mouth, face, neck, trunk, arms, and legs.

Medical history included aortic stenosis and osteoarthritis. There was no personal or family history of neurologic illness or of alcohol or drug abuse. Her physical exam was normal for her age except for a Grade III/IV systolic ejection murmur and involuntary movements. Mental status exam showed normal mood and affect, with no delusions, hallucinations, or formal thought disorder. Insight and judgment were adequate, and her Mini-Mental State Exam score was 28/30. Her AIMS score was 22, indicating the severity of her TD.

The patient then consented to participate in a series of placebo-controlled, double-blind drug trials of 3 months each. She failed to show any improvement with choline chloride (18 g/day), sodium valproate (2500 mg/day), 5-hydroxytryptophan (400 mg/day with carbidopa 100 mg/day), and L-dopa (400 mg/day with carbidopa 100 mg/day), but showed noticeable but partial improvement with the dopamine synthesis inhibitor alpha-methylparatyrosine (AMPT) (3000 mg/day). However, her movements worsened after 2 weeks on AMPT.

Two years after admission, and after having finished the above series of drug trials, the patient's abnormal movements were essentially unchanged.

The patient was then given a trial of EST recommended by her referring physician, mainly for her severe osteoporosis, but monitoring of her tardive dyskinesia continued. She received Premarin at a dosage of 1.25 mg/day. Within 2 months, there was a marked decrease in her AIMS score (down to 14) and after a total of 4 months, her movements had further decreased (AIMS score of 9). The improvement was apparent in all areas: facial, orobuccal, truncal, and peripheral. The patient seemed considerably relaxed and relieved, and her friends and relatives all agreed that she was better than ever before. A 1-year follow-up showed that the patient was still doing well, and had returned to her favorite hobbies of needle work and crochet, which she had had to give up several years before.

This case of severe and persistent tardive dyskinesia that failed to respond to a series of controlled interventions showed a remarkable and gratifying degree of improvement with EST. The use of EST treatment in postmenopausal patients with severe and persistent tardive dyskinesia should be considered.

PROLACTIN, STRIATAL DOPAMINE, AND TD

In the studies of TD patients described above it appears that elevated PRL levels correlated with TD severity in hypoestrogenic women. Such an observation suggests that PRL itself could play a role in the pathogenesis of TD.

Animal studies have reported that peptide and protein hormones usually thought to originate from the pituitary have been detected within the central nervous system by a number of techniques (40, 41). Hokfelt et al. (42) demonstrated PRL-like immunoreactivity localized in the nerve terminals of rat hypothalamus. Walsh et al. (43) used a competitive binding assay in combination with microscopic autoradiography to demonstrate PRL binding sites in the hypothalamus and choroid plexes of the rat. Following up Fuxe et al.'s work, Toubeau et al. (44–46) used an antiserum to PRL to identify PRL-containing neurons and fibers in intact and hypophysectomized female rats. PRL has been shown to increase DA turnover and secretion in the tuberoinfundibular DA tract (47–49). Although PRL binding sites have not been identified in the striatum, several studies in rats have reported that hypophysectomy abolishes the effects of EST on striatal DA function (29, 50–52).

Following these observations, other investigators (53) reported an effect of EST on DA function independent of PRL. It has been suggested that this discrepancy is due to sexual differentiation of the mechanism by which EST changes striatal DA function (25). Nevertheless, it appears that when PRL levels are increased, DA receptor density increases in both male and ovariectomized female rats (25). In addition, in the study of midbrain-lesioned ovariectomized monkeys reported above (36), domperidone, the peripheral dopamine antagonist, was given in a dose of 1 mg/kg intramuscularly. Similar to the effect of estradiol, domperidone, which elevates PRL levels without crossing the blood–brain barrier, caused an inhibition of apomorphine-exacerbated dyskinesia at 24 hours and a facilitation at 3 days to 2 weeks. The basic data remain unclear but may ultimately help explain the clinical observation of a positive association between baseline hyperprolactinemia and severity of TD in postmenopausal females. It is possible that the loss of EST in women with high PRL values (presumably from chronic antipsychotic medication exposure) renders them vulnerable to increased severity of TD. We speculate that the PRL itself could contribute to the severity of TD through striatal DA mechanisms. An ideal strategy to test this hypothesis in humans would involve treating TD by lowering PRL levels. Unfortunately, there is no agent that will act on the pituitary without also acting on the striatum or other central nervous system DA systems.

CONCLUSION

Neuroendocrine themes must be considered in studies of the pathogenesis of TD. Basic and clinical studies point to the importance of considering how EST and PRL influence DA function in the brain. Animal studies suggest that EST and PRL, separately or in concert, affect striatal DA function via a neurotransmitter, or more likely a neuromodulator's mechanism. There is some evidence suggesting that menopause is a risk factor for TD occurrence. Studies of TD patients have shown that 1) hyperprolactinemia correlates with TD severity in hypoestrogenic women, 2) plasma HVA correlates with TD severity in postmenopausal women but not men, and 3) EST replacement therapy improves TD severity in postmenopausal women. It should be kept in mind that EST could be involved in the mechanisms underlying some cases of TD by exerting 1) a central direct or indirect (via the pituitary) effect on striatal DA; 2) a peripheral effect, for example, altering the metabolism or distribution of DA-related medication (26, 54–58), or 3) a central effect via a nondopaminergic system such as serotonin or gamma-aminobutyric acid that affects the striatum.

These data have implications for future research involving the epidemiology and pharmacology of TD. If possible, menopause status should be included as an important clinical variable and considered as a predictor of TD severity or occurrence. Determining menopause status in neuroleptic-treated women can be problematic because amenorrhea is a common consequence of this treatment. However, careful attention to the other signs and symptoms associated with menopause will help in this regard (59).

The neuroendocrine themes discussed in this chapter demonstrate how the field of psychiatry has evolved to the point where it must work in concert with data from the basic neurosciences. It is hoped that this chapter stimulates further collaboration between clinicians and laboratory scientists in this exciting area.

REFERENCES

1. Klawans H: The pharmacology of tardive dyskinesia. Am J Psychiatry 1973

2. Balthazart J, Prove E, Gilles R: Hormones and Behavior in Higher Vertebrates. New York, Springer-Verlag, 1983

3. Jeste D, Wyatt R: Therapeutic strategies against tardive dyskinesia. Arch Gen Psychiatry 29:803–816, 1982

4. Smith JM, Baldessarini RJ: Changes in prevalence, severity and recovery in tardive dyskinesia with age. Arch Gen Psychiatry 37:1368–1373, 1980

5. Jus A, Peneau R, Lachance R: The epidemiology of tardive dyskinesia. Part I. Dis Nerv Syst 33:182–186, 1976

6. Kennedy PF, Hershon HI, McGuire RJ: Extrapyramidal disorders after prolonged phenothiazine therapy. Br J Psychiatry 118:509–518, 1971

7. Smith JM, Oswald WT, Kucharski LT: Tardive dyskinesia: age and sex differences in hospitalized schizophrenics. Psychopharmacol 58:207–211, 1978

8. Kleinbert DL, Noel GL, Grantz AG: Chlorpromazine stimulation and L-dopa suppression of plasma prolactin in man. J Clin Endocrinol Metab 33:873–875, 1971

9. Sachar EJ, Gruen PH, Altman N, et al: Use of neuroendocrine techniques in psychopharmacologic research, in Hormones, Behavior and Psychopathology. Edited by Sachar EJ. New York, Raven Press, 1976, pp. 161–176

10. Meltzer HY, So R, Miller RJ, et al: Comparison of the effects of substituted benzamides and standard neuroleptics on the binding of ^{3}H-spiroperidol in the rat pituitary and striatum with in vivo effects on rat prolactin secretion. Life Sci 25:573–584, 1979

11. Glazer WM, Moore DC, Bowers MB, et al: Serum prolactin and tardive dyskinesia. Am J Psychiatry 138:1493–1496, 1981

12. Glazer W, Moore DC: The diagnosis of rapid abnormal involuntary movements associated with fluphenazine decanoate. J Nerv Ment Dis 168:439–441, 1980

13. Glazer WM: Notes from a tardive dyskinesia clinic. Yale Psychiatric Quarterly 8:4–15, 1986

14. Beumont PJ, Corker CS, Kriesen HG: The effects of phenothiazines on endocrine function, II. Br J Psychiatry 124:420–430, 1974

15. McEwen BS, Davis PG, Parsons B: The brain as a target for steroid hormone action. Ann Rev Neurosci 2:65–112, 1979

16. Pfaff D, Keiner M: Atlas of estradiol concentrating cells in the central nervous system of the female rat. J Compar Neurol 51:121–158, 1973

17. Stumpf WE, Sar M, Keefer DA: Atlas of estrogen target cells in rat brain, in Anatomical Neuroendocrinology. Edited by Stumpf WE, Grant LD. Switzerland, Karger Press, 1975, pp. 104–119

18. Heritage AS, Stumpf WE, Sar M, et al: Brainstem catecholamine neurons are target sites for sex steroid hormones. Science 207:1377–1378, 1980

19. Kelly MJ, Moss RL, Dudley CA, et al: The specificity of the response of preoptic-septal area neurons to estrogen: 17a estradiol versus 17b estradiol and the response of extrahypothalamic neurons. Exp Brain Res 30:43–52, 1977

20. Mueller E, Nistico G, Scapagnini V: Neurotransmitters and Anterior Pituitary Function. New York, Academic Press, 1977

21. Bedard P, Boucher R, Di Paolo T, et al: Biphasic effect of estradiol and domperidone on lingual dyskinesia in monkeys. Exp Neurol 82:172–182, 1983.

22. Villeneuve A, Cazejust T, Cote M: Estrogens in tardive dyskinesia in male psychiatric patients. Neuropsychobiology 6:145–151, 1980

23. Zegart KN, Schwarz RH: Chorea gravidarum. Obstet Gynecol 32:24–27, 1968

24. Nausieda PA, Koller WC, Weiner WJ, et al: Modification of post-synaptic dopaminergic sensitivity by female sex hormones. Life Sci 25:521–526, 1979

25. Hruska RE: Sex hormone exposure and nonreproductive behavior. Int J Ment Health 14:112–134, 1985

26. Chiodo LA, Caggiula AR, Saller CF: Estrogen increases both spiperone-induced catalepsy and brain levels of [^{3}H] spiperone in the rat. Brain Res 172:360–366, 1979

27. Bueno J, Pfaff DW: Single unit recording in hypothalamus and preoptic area of estrogen-treated and untreated ovariectomized female rats. Brain Res 101:67–78, 1976

28. Chiodo LA, Caggiula AR: Alterations in basal firing rate and auto-receptor sensitivity of dopamine neurons in the substantia nigra following acute and extended exposure to estrogen. Eur J Pharmacol 67:165–166, 1980

29. Arnauld E, Dufy B, Pestre M, et al: Effects of estrogens on the responses of caudate neurons to microiontophoretically applied dopamine. Neurosci Lett 21:325–331, 1981

30. Chiodo LA, Caggiula AR: Substantia nigral dopamine neurons: alterations in basal discharge rates and autoreceptor sensitivity induced by estrogen. Neuropharmacol 22:593–599, 1983

31. Chiodo LA, Glazer WM, Bunney BS: Midbrain dopamine neurons: electrophysiological studies on the acute effects of estrogen in Dopaminergic Systems and Their Regulation, Edited by Woodruff GN, Poat JA, Roberts PG. London, MacMillan Press, 1986, pp. 303–311

32. Bell RC, Smith RC: Tardive dyskinesia: characterization and prevalence in a statewide system. J Clin Psychiatry 39:39–47, 1978

33. Glazer, WM, Naftolin F, Moore DC, et al: The relationship of circulating estradiol to tardive dyskinesia in men and postmenopausal women. Psychoneuroendocrinology 8:429–434, 1983

34. Gordon JH, Diamond BI: Antagonism of dopamine supersensitivity by estrogen: neurochemical studies in an animal model of tardive dyskinesia. Biol Psychiatry 16:365–371, 1981

35. Fields JZ, Gordon JH: Estrogen inhibits the dopaminergic supersensitivity induced by neuroleptics. Life Sci 30:229–234, 1982

36. Bedard P, Boucher R, Di Paolo T, et al: Biphasic effect of estradiol and domperidone on lingual dyskinesia in monkeys. Exp Neurol 82:172–182, 1983

37. Glazer WM, Naftolin F, Morgenstern H, et al: Estrogen replacement and tardive dyskinesia. Psychoneuroendocrinology 10:345–350, 1985

38. Weiss NS, Szekely DR, Austin DF: Increasing incidence of endometrial cancer in the United States. N Eng J Med 294:1259–1262, 1976

39. MacDonald PC: Estrogen plus progestin in postmenopausal women—ACT II. N Engl J Med 315:959–961, 1986

40. Krieger, DT, Liotta AS: Pituitary hormones in brain: where, how and why? Science 61:13–16, 1979

41. Fuxe K, Hokfelt T, Eneroth P: Prolactin: localization in nerve terminals of the rat hypothalamus. Science 196:899–908, 1977

42. Hokfelt T, Elde R, Fuxe K, et al: Aminergic and peptidergic pathways in the nervous system with special reference to the hypothalamus, in The Hypothalamus. Edited by Reichlin S, Baldessarini RJ, Martin JB. New York, Raven Press, 1978, pp. 69–135

43. Walsh R, Bosner B, Kopriwa B, et al: Prolactin binding sites in the rat brain. Science 201:1041–1042, 1978

44. Tobeau G, Desclin J, Parmentier M, et al: Compared localizations of prolactin-like and adrenocorticotropin immunoreactivities within the brain of the rat. Neuroendocrinology 29:374–384, 1979

45. Tobeau G, Desclin J, Parmentier M, et al: Cellular localization of a prolactin-like antigen in the rat brain. J Endocrinol 83:261–266, 1979

46. Tobeau G, Desclin J, Parmentier M, et al: Identification of a prolactin-like peptide in rat hypothalamic neurons. Annales D Endrinologie 41:137–138, 1980

47. Annunziato L, Moore KE: Prolactin CSH selectively increases dopamine turnover in the median eminence. Life Sci 22:2037–2042, 1978

48. Cramer OM, Parker CR, Porter JC: Secretion of dopamine into hypophysial portal blood by rats bearing prolactin-secreting or ectopic pituitary glands. Endocrinology 105:526–529, 1979

49. Gudelsky GA, Porter JC: Release of dopamine from tuberoinfundibular neurons into pituitary stalk blood after prolactin or haloperidol administration. Endocrinology 106:526–529, 1980

50. Euvrard C, Labrie F, Boissier JR: Effect of moxestrol on haloperidol-induced changes in striatal acetylcholine levels and dopamine turnover. Comm Psychopharm 3:329–339, 1979

51. Euvrard C, Labrie F, Boissier JR: Effect of estrogen on changes in the activity of striatal cholinergic neurons induced by DA drugs. Brain Res 169:215–220, 1979

52. Kumakura K, Hoffman M, Cocchi D, et al: Long-term effects of ovariectomy on dopamine-stimulated adenylate cyclase in rat striatum and nucleus accumbens. Psychopharmacology 61:13–16, 1979

53. Di Paolo T, Daigle M, Labrie F: Effect of estradiol and haloperidol on hypophysectomized rat brain dopamine receptors. Psychoneuroendocrinology 9:399–404, 1984

54. Chiodo LA, Caggiula AR, Saller CF: Estrogen potentiates the stereotypy induced by dopamine agonists in the rat. Life Sci 28:827–835, 1981

55. Cooney A: Environmental factors influencing drug metabolism in Fundamentals of Drug Metabolism and Drug Disposition. Edited by LaDu BN, Mandel HG, Way E. Baltimore, Williams and Wilkins, 1971, pp. 253–278

56. Lal S, Sourkes THL: Potentiation and inhibition of the amphetamine stereotypy in rats by neuroleptics and other agents. Arch Int Pharmacodyn Ther 199:298–301, 1972

57. Kato R: Sex related differences in drug metabolism. Drug Metab Rev 3:1–32, 1974

58. DeFrewy EL, Marsy S, Mannering G: Sex dependent differences in drug metabolism in the rat II. Qualitative change produced by castration and the administration of steroid hormones and pentobarbital. Drug Metab Dis 2:279–284, 1974

59. Ballinger CB: Psychiatric morbidity and the menopause: survey of a gynecological out-patient clinic. Br J Psychiatry 131:83–89, 1977

Chapter 14

Pathophysiology and Therapy of Tardive Dyskinesia: The GABA Connection

Gunvant K. Thaker, M.D.
Thomas N. Ferraro, Ph.D.
Theodore A. Hare, Ph.D.
Carol A. Tamminga, M.D.

Chapter 14

Pathophysiology and Therapy of Tardive Dyskinesia: The GABA Connection

The involuntary motor disorder called tardive dyskinesia (TD), which occurs as a late consequence of chronic neuroleptic treatment, presents a formidable problem for psychiatric research (1). Its pathophysiology remains unexplained, and treatments do not exist. While dopamine (DA) receptor supersensitivity has traditionally been cited as the putative mechanism underlying the motor disorder (2), it is now thought to be an inadequate explanation. On the basis of several lines of reported evidence, and our own experimental data, we propose that the major inhibitory transmitter system in the basal ganglia, gamma-aminobutyric acid (GABA), is dysfunctional in some chronically neuroleptic-treated patients, resulting in TD. More specifically, basic research suggests that, whereas all mammalian brains treated chronically with neuroleptic drugs develop DA receptor supersensitivity in striatum (3, 4), only some go on to develop abnormalities in GABA-mediated transmission in the substantia nigra pars reticulata (5), a primary projection field of the striatum. Since this nucleus collects and projects information from the entire basal ganglia to the thalamus and brainstem (6–10), any dysfunction occurring here has broad functional implications. Both clinical and preclinical evidence is reviewed in this chapter to examine the pharmacological, biochemical, and neurophysiological role of GABA neuronal system function in TD. If, indeed, a GABA system abnormality is the determinant of TD, then treatment can be focused on that transmitter system, and its potential diagnostic, predictive, and prophylactic power for TD can be explored.

Neuroleptics are now universally used for acute and maintenance treatment of schizophrenia. Meanwhile, TD, the late-emerging choreoathetoid side effect, has been recognized in 20 to 25 percent of chronically treated patients and threatens the continued use of neuroleptics in this group. Currently, two decades after the recognition of this side effect, a precise understanding of its pathophysiology and a definitive treatment for the disorder are still lacking. Development of supersensitive DA receptors has been the traditional hypothesis used to explain the disorder (2, 11–13). This is based on evidence of the proliferation of DA receptors and an increase in their affinity with chronic neuroleptic treatment. DA agonist drugs increase (14) and DA antagonists decrease (15–17) the hyperkinetic symptoms in TD, thus supporting a DA supersensitivity hypothesis of TD. However, direct evidence for this supersensitivity hypothesis is lacking: DA metabolites in cerebrospinal fluid (CSF) (18) and postmortem brain, DA receptor binding in postmortem tissue (19, 20), and DA-mediated endocrinological measurements (21) fail to show differences between TD and non-TD patients. Inconsistencies like coexistence of both dyskinetic and parkinsonian symptoms in the same body region are difficult to explain by the DA hypothesis. And, most significantly, both experimental animal and human postmortem studies reveal an overall development of supersensitive DA receptors in brain with chronic neuroleptic treatment (3, 4, 19, 20), whereas only a fraction of chronically treated patients manifest TD. This suggests that in addition to the supersensitivity of DA receptors, other factors are likely to play a determinant role in the emergence of TD.

BASAL GANGLIA GABA NEURONAL SYSTEM

Gamma-aminobutyric acid (GABA) is a major inhibitory neurotransmitter located throughout brain, including the basal ganglia (22); here it mediates both intrinsic and major efferent neuronal pathways (6). DA and GABA interact in several ways in the basal ganglia. First, there exists a GABA-mediated striatonigral pathway that provides a negative "feedback loop" to modulate nigral DA cell activity (23, 24). This regulation is provided by branching collaterals of the striatonigral GABAergic neurons that terminate mainly in pars reticulata and influence the DA neurons through a GABAergic interneuron. Second, the striatonigral neurons predominantly influence a set of substantia nigra reticulata (SNR) GABAergic neurons, forming a major nigral efferent pathway to thalamus, superior colliculus, and reticular formation (8, 9, 25). An increase in the activity of pars compacta dopaminergic cells, through striatal interneuron (cholinergic or GABAergic), serves to increase activity in the striatonigral GABAergic neurons (6), which in turn inhibits the tonic firing of nigral GABAergic efferents (6, 7).

The nigral efferents project to intermediate and deep layers of the superior colliculus (SC), ventral medial and ventral lateral nuclei of thalamus, and the brainstem reticular formation (8). There is a rich collateral system among these efferents. Experimentally, most of the motor behavior associated with DA receptor stimulation or blockade can be reproduced or antagonized by appropriate manipulation of these GABAergic efferents in laboratory animals. For instance, unilateral muscimol (GABA$_A$ agonist) injected into the SNR of a rat produces contralateral turning behavior (26, 27), and bilateral muscimol injected into SNR can produce stereotypied or hyperkinetic movements in the experimental animals (28–30). These GABAergic actions are thought to be independent of the DA pathway since the pharmacologic probe is injected locally and haloperidol treatment does not block the effect. Furthermore, brain hemitransection in rat just rostral to the substantia nigra produces an animal preparation that still retains these GABA-related activities (31–33).

Chronic neuroleptic treatment has been shown to alter GABA neuronal activity in the basal ganglia. It produces a decrease in GABA concentration and loss of activity of the GABA synthesizing enzyme, glutamic acid decarboxylase (GAD), in the SNR of laboratory animals (5, 7, 34–36). Also, an increase in the number of GABA binding sites in the substantia nigra has been found in rats and an increase in the sensitivity of behavioral electrophysiologic responses to a muscimol challenge has been observed in animals treated chronically with neuroleptics (37, 38). Other methods of striatal DA denervation like 6-hydroxydopamine (6-OHDA) lesions of the nigrostriatal dopaminergic pathway or kainic acid lesions of the striatonigral pathways also produce supersensitive GABA receptors in the substantia nigra (39, 40).

These changes in the GABA system with chronic neuroleptic treatment seem to be dyskinesia specific in primates. Gunne et al. (5) treated monkeys with neuroleptics for 22 to 26 years and some of them developed dyskinetic movements. Postmortem evaluation of the animals suggested significant reduction in GAD activity and GABA levels in the substantia nigra of monkeys who developed dyskinesia compared to nondyskinetic or nontreated control monkeys. These findings are of particular significance with regard to the pathophysiology of TD, since loss of GABAergic input to the substantia nigra has been shown to produce transneuronal death of nigral neurons in the rat (41). Neuronal destruction of the SNR or bilateral inhibition of SNR efferents can produce stereotypied and hyperkinetic movements in animals (42, 43).

In summary, nigral GABA neuronal activity appears to play a

pivotal role in the modulation of basal ganglia function. Inhibition or disruption of these tonically firing GABA-mediated nigral efferents produces hyperkinetic movements in animals. Chronic neuroleptic treatment produces alterations in the nigral GABA system including supersensitivity of GABA receptors located on neurons of nigral GABAergic efferents. On the basis of the above rationale, we have developed the hypothesis that alterations in the nigral GABA system may play a critical role in the pathophysiology of TD.

Direct testing of this hypothesis in human patients has remained difficult. However, indirect evidence derived from GABA pharmacology in TD has accumulated. In addition, we have evaluated cerebrospinal fluid (CSF) biochemistry as a measure of the activity of central GABAergic transmission. We have also studied the functional significance of GABA abnormality in basal ganglia by testing oculomotor performance, based on the known role of GABAergic efferents from the basal ganglia in mediating saccades (44, 45). Results from such a neurophysiological study carried out in TD patients are presented to support the GABA hypothesis of TD.

CLINICAL PHARMACOLOGY OF GABAMIMETICS IN TD

GABA agonist drugs appear to be therapeutic in TD, and various lines of preclinical evidence, many of which have already been reviewed, support this. However, the GABA-mimetic strategy in TD has been confounded in its development by two major problems. First, systemic GABA-mimetic drug administration could have opposing actions in brain, since GABA mediates multiple neuronal pathways in basal ganglia at least some of which are linked in a series (10, 46). Whereas striatonigral GABAergic neurons are phasic in their activity, nigral efferents provide a tonic inhibitory signal to the terminal areas. Disruption of these efferent pathways and the subsequent tonic disinhibition of terminal areas is hypothesized to play a role in the pathophysiology of TD. Systemic GABAergic treatment may act preferentially at the terminal areas that are normally tonically inhibited and where the "deficit" is present. Even though the GABAergic treatment may preferentially act at this site of "deficit," complete remission of the dyskinetic symptoms may still be difficult to achieve.

Second, specific antidyskinetic effects of GABA-mimetic drugs without any untoward side effects have been difficult to achieve. This may be because GABA is so ubiquitous and multifunctional in the brain. However, since different subtypes of GABA receptors are now thought to exist (47), a receptor-specific drug may have increased functional specificity, thus augmenting the utility of GABA-mimetic drug therapy in disease states like TD. At present, GABA$_A$ and GABA$_B$ subtypes of receptors are well described in the literature (48), GABA$_A$ is a bicuculline-sensitive receptor associated with chloride channels; muscimol and tetrahydroisoxazolopyridinol (THIP) are specifically active at this site. On the other hand, the GABA$_B$ receptor is insensitive to bicuculline, is associated with calcium channels, and has baclofen as a specific ligand. Progabide and GABA are mixed GABA$_A$ and GABA$_B$ agonists. Although both subtypes of GABA receptor are distributed in basal ganglia and related areas, clinical data suggest that GABA$_A$ agonists may be more effective antidyskinetic agents.

CLINICAL TRIALS WITH GABAERGIC DRUGS IN TD

Early GABA Mimetics. Drugs like sodium valproate and baclofen were tested for antidyskinetic activity in the 1970s. Inconsistent antidyskinetic effects that were observed with their use may be explained by the weak, if any, central GABA-mimetic actions of sodium valproate at the clinical doses tested. In addition, baclofen is now known to act only at subpopulation of GABA receptors, namely, the GABA$_B$ receptors (49).

GABA$_A$ Receptor Agonists. The first clinical trial of a specific GABA$_A$ agonist drug was carried out in 1979 in seven neuroleptic-free schizophrenic patients with moderate to severe TD (50). In a placebo-controlled trial, muscimol was administered in doses up to 9 mg/day to young schizophrenic patients with moderate to severe TD. A significant (48 percent) decrease in dyskinetic symptoms was observed during the muscimol treatment. Another GABA analog, THIP, active at GABA$_A$ receptor sites, was evaluated in 13 patients with dyskinesias (51). In contrast to the muscimol study, patients were older (mean age 61 years; four patients were over 70 years of age), and some carried a diagnosis of dementia and were concurrently receiving neuroleptic treatment. While only three participants received THIP at doses up to 120 mg/day, the majority of the patients received the drug in doses up to 20–90 mg/day. No decrease in dyskinesias was observed in this group of patients; a minimal increase in preexisting parkinsonian symptoms and a decrease in eye-blink rate were noted at the maximum doses. Side effects such as confusion, vomiting, dizziness, and sedation were common, disallowing use of higher doses in the majority of participants.

In a more recent double-blind placebo-controlled trial, we administered THIP to two neuroleptic-free TD patients (52). Participants received up to 120 mg and 60 mg each of THIP. A slight (35 percent) but consistent dose-dependent antidyskinetic effect was observed in both patients. Side effects such as episodic mental status changes and withdrawal-induced seizures precluded further use of the drug. This mild antidyskinetic action of THIP in these two studies may be due to the fact that the drug is active only at a subpopulation of GABA receptors (53).

Progabide is another GABA-mimetic drug, active at the $GABA_A$ and $GABA_B$ receptors and available for clinical testing. Encouraged by positive results in a preliminary open study in 19 neuroleptic-treated patients (54), Morselli et al. (55) repeated the progabide trial in a double-blind design in 10 patients. Patients were on stable neuroleptic dose and received 900 to 1200 mg of progabide for 6 weeks. The preliminary report from this group indicates a significant (60 percent) reduction in the mean dyskinesia score during this progabide treatment. We have also been testing the antidyskinetic action of progabide administered for 5 weeks at doses of 45 mg/kg in a double-blind, placebo-controlled randomized cross-over trial. Preliminary results from three neuroleptic-free patients are available (56). A significant and moderate decrease (on average 40 percent) in dyskinetic symptoms with the progabide treatment has been noted consistently in all three patients.

GABA-Transaminase Inhibitors. Gamma-acetylenic GABA (GAG) and the gamma-vinyl GABA (GVG) are two effective irreversible catalytic inhibitors of GABA-transaminase (57, 58). While GVG may be more specific in its actions, both drugs raise brain GABA levels (56, 60) in laboratory animal tissue and humans (CSF).

GAG was tested in 10 psychiatric patients, 7 with schizophrenia, 2 with organic brain syndrome and 1 with manic–depressive illness; 4 patients were treated concurrently with multiple neuroleptics and anticholinergics and 2 were on lithium (61). On average, a 33 percent decrease in dyskinetic symptoms was noted; however, in two elderly patients there was an increase and in one (with organic dementia) there was no change in symptoms.

Four independent groups have used GVG in doses from 3 to 6 g/day in TD (62–65). Tell et al. (62) reported a significant dose-related improvement in seven of their nine TD patients with GVG treatment up to 6 g/day. Interestingly, two patients with senile dementia experienced an increase in their dyskinetic symptoms. Similar but perhaps more encouraging results were obtained in a double-blind cross-over study in neuroleptic-free, younger (mean ± SD = 28.7 ± 4.5, range = 22 to 36 years) schizophrenic patients with TD (63). All patients were able to tolerate GVG doses up to 3 g. Significant reductions of 44 percent in dyskinesias were observed during the GVG treatment compared to both pretrial baseline and placebo treatment periods. Interestingly, the antidyskinetic effect paralleled a robust (>100 percent) increase in lumbar CSF GABA but not in 32 other amino acids that were measured (64). No major side effects, including parkinsonian symptoms and sedation, or any laboratory abnormality was noted.

Korsgaard et al. (65) used GVG in doses up to 2 g (four patients) and 6 g (six patients) in individuals concurrently treated with neuroleptic drugs. The authors reported a moderate (39 percent) antidyskinetic response in seven patients associated with an increase in preexisting parkinsonian side effects. No effect on psychoses was noted, but confusion (two participants), mild sedation (in three; moderate in one) and dizziness (one patient) were observed. Another GVG study (66) was performed in nine patients with mixed diagnoses (seven with TD, one each with Meige's and Tourette's syndromes). Patients were concurrently on chronic stable neuroleptic dose. Overall, there was a significant antidyskinetic effect in TD; in four patients there was a clinically significant improvement. The two patients with a dyskinesia diagnosis different from TD did not respond.

In conclusion, six reports and three preliminary sets of data regarding specific GABAergic treatments in TD are available for review. A total of 78 patients with TD participated in these studies; 56 (72 percent) of them responded to the GABA-mimetic treatment. The average response in these studies ranged from 28 to 60 percent. This was a clinically significant reduction in TD.

To evaluate the reasons for nonresponse to the GABA-mimetic drugs, we divided the total number of participants reported in these studies into GABA agonist responders and nonresponders (50, 55, 61–64). Patient description was not available in 10 patients (all were responders), leaving a total sample of 68 for analysis. Out of these, 46 patients responded to GABA mimetics and 22 did not. We compared these two groups on demographic variables including age, diagnoses, and gender. Although presence of concurrent neuroleptics may be an important variable, it was not used for comparison because few experimental subjects were off neuroleptics. As can be seen in Table 1, individuals who failed to respond to GABA-mimetic treatment were older and more frequently carried a diagnosis of dementia. This suggests that the involuntary movements in this older group are pathophysiologically different from those in young persons and possibly related to dementia. Furthermore, the drug pharmacodynamics and the existing neuronal functional status might be different in these elderly, demented patients, thus potentially explaining greater frequency of treatment failures.

Table 1. Comparison of patient's characteristics between GABA responders and GABA nonresponders

Patients	Mean age (years) ± SD	Duration of tardive dyskinesia in years	Diagnosis of dementia
GABA responders[a] (n = 46)	43.9 ± 18.3	4.3 ± 4.4	2/46
GABA nonresponders[b] (n = 22)	60.2 ± 13.2*	4.6 ± 4.4	6/22†

[a]Participants from the Morselli et al. (55) study were not included (n = 10, all responders) since demographic information was not available.
[b]In the Korsgaard et al. (51) study, all 13 patients are presumed to be nonresponders since it was a negative study. However, the response of each individual participant is not known. If this study is excluded, then the mean age of nonresponders becomes even higher.
*$p < 0.001$ by Student's t test.
†$p < 0.02$ by Fisher's exact test.

Direct GABA Agonist: Side Effects. Untoward effects were troublesome in many of these studies with GABA-mimetic drugs. Muscimol is known to be psychotomimetic and has a low therapeutic/toxic ratio; GAG and THIP were also associated with numerous untoward effects. Progabide was found to be associated with liver toxicity in a significant minority of patients. GVG was one of the least toxic GABAergic drugs; unfortunately, due to microvacuolization observed in white matter of rat, the drug is currently unavailable for further clinical studies (65). On reviewing the clinical trials of GABAergic drugs, one may infer that side effects such as sedation, confusion, dizziness, and myoclonic jerks are more common when the GABA-mimetic drug is used in combination with neuroleptics or other centrally active drugs. Furthermore, an association between an increase in preexisting parkinsonian symptoms and a decrease in dyskinesias was reported in two studies. However, the existence of a significant association does not necessarily mean a causal effect, and other evidence supports a conclusion to the contrary; for example, many studies show an antidyskinetic effect without parkinsonian effect and one negative study observed a slight increase in parkinsonian symptoms. When these drugs are used in neuroleptic-free subjects emergence of parkinsonian symptoms is not observed, suggesting that although they have an observable antidyskinetic action, the GABAergic drugs by themselves do not cause parkinsonian symptoms at the clinical doses used.

GABA Function Enhancers: Benzodiazepines. In contrast to the above specific GABAergic drugs, benzodiazepines (BZD) are available for clinical use and have few toxic effects. Some BZD receptors are known to be linked with $GABA_A$ receptors to form GABA-BZD-chloride ionophore (66). Through an action on opening the chloride ion channels, BZD potentiates the effect of GABA on $GABA_A$ receptors (67). Review of the literature shows that BZDs are modestly effective as antidyskinetic agents (68). Eighty-five percent of the total 154 TD patients in these reports moderately responded to the BZD treatment. We have evaluated clonazepam in doses up to 2–4 mg/day for 4 weeks as an add-on treatment in chronic neuroleptic-treated schizophrenic patients with TD (n = 19) in a double-blind, placebo-controlled, randomized cross-over design. On average, a 35 percent decrease in dyskinetic symptoms was observed during clonazepam treatment compared to placebo (p < 0.01). Sedation was observed in six patients, dizziness and hypotension in one, and ataxia in three individuals. Dose reduction allowed further use of the drug without any side effects. Unfortunately, in the subsequent open study, gradual development of tolerance to the effect was observed over 20 to 30 weeks and this may limit the clinical utility of BZD. But, clonazepam can be used clinically for up to a year in many patients selected because of severe symptoms and demonstrate good response to the drug. Tolerance to the antidyskinetic effect can be managed to some extent by including a 1- to 2-week clonazepam-free period in their long-term treatment.

The above review shows that augmenting central GABA activity directly by receptor stimulation or indirectly by receptor potentiation or degradatory enzyme inhibition, all decrease dyskinetic symptoms. Besides the obvious therapeutic significance of these findings, the pharmacological data are consistent with the idea that reduced GABA activity in critical areas of brain may play a pathophysiologic role in TD. To further explore this hypothesis we carried out CSF GABA measurements in drug-free schizophrenic patients with TD in comparison with those without TD.

CSF NEUROCHEMISTRY

Analysis of various monoamines and their metabolites in CSF has been frequently carried out to explore the neurochemical basis of TD (18, 69). No significant changes in dopaminergic or other monoaminergic metabolite levels are observed in the CSF of TD patients (69).

CSF GABA is thought to be mainly derived from the cerebral tissue (70). GABA does not penetrate the blood–brain barrier (71), and a rostro-caudal gradient exists (72). Further, changes in brain GABA activity in disease conditions (for example, Huntington's chorea) have been found to be reflected in the CSF GABA levels (70). Similarly, increases in the brain GABA concentrations in animals following central pharmacological GABA-T inhibition produces corresponding increases in CSF GABA levels (73). Therefore, to evaluate brain GABA activity we measured CSF GABA levels in schizophrenic patients with and without TD.

All the participants were at least 4 weeks drug free. Patients were matched by age and psychiatric diagnoses. Mean age of TD patients was 26.6 years (SD = ± 3.9, range = 22 to 32 years), and of non-TD patients was 27.4 years (SD = ± 3.5, range = 22 to 31). Both groups were identical with respect to variables such as total duration of neuroleptic treatment, total scores on the Brief Psychiatric Rating Scale and its subscales, and duration of psychiatric illness. Lumbar spinal fluid was collected on ice by standard technique. The first 13 ml of CSF were mixed together and separated into 1 ml samples for immediate freezing and storage. Such a technique of collection and handling avoids posttap artifactual increases in GABA levels (74). Samples from all the patients were analyzed in the same batch at a later date. High performance liquid chromatography (HPLC)-ion-exchange fluorometric technique was used as a GABA assay (75). A significant decrease in CSF GABA levels was observed in schizophrenic patients with TD compared to those without. There was a negative correlation between the amount of dyskinesia and CSF GABA levels (Pearson's r = − 0.44, p = 0.06). None of the other clinical variables showed a significant correlation with the CSF GABA.

The above findings suggest that TD in schizophrenic patients is associated with a lowered CSF GABA. This provides indirect evidence to support the hypothesis that there is a decrease in brain GABA activity in TD. Although the preclinical, especially the primate, studies would localize this deficit in basal ganglia, CSF GABA levels cannot localize the GABA change to basal ganglia activity. However, to further investigate the role of the basal ganglia GABAergic pathways in TD, one can explore the functional behavioral "markers" of these GABA efferent pathways in TD.

OCULOMOTOR NEUROPHYSIOLOGY

The superior colliculus along with thalamus and brainstem reticular formation are the terminal areas of nigral projections. The GABAergic efferent from SNR represents one of the most prominent inputs to the intermediate and deep layers of SC. The nigrotectal pathway tonically inhibits collicular cells involved in the generation of saccadic eye movements. When primates are presented with a visual stimuli, there is a "pause" in the tonic firing of nigral cells, thus disinhibiting the collicular neurons and allowing initiation of a saccade. Complete disruption of these nigrotectal pathways in the experimental monkey produces increased saccadic "distractibility"; monkeys fixate poorly and often fail to inhibit inappropriate saccades toward a "distracting" stimuli. We have previously reported a similar increase in "distractibility" of saccadic system in schizophrenic patients with tardive dyskinesia (76).

Twenty-five schizophrenic patients (15 with and 10 without TD) and eight normals consented to participate in the eye movement study. Subjects were matched by age (mean ± SD = 34.2 ± 6.1, 33.7 ± 5.8, and 30.13 ± 3.04 years for TD, non-TD, and normal subjects, respectively). Patients were taking chronic neuroleptic treatment at chlorpromazine equivalent doses of 1857 ± 2453 mg and 1198 ± 1578 mg per day for TD and non-TD groups, respectively. Eye movements were measured by an electrooculogram method to evaluate saccadic latency and distractibility in two experimental paradigms. In the first paradigm, subjects were instructed to look at the target, whereas in the second experiment, subjects were instructed to look away from the distracting stimuli. Inappropriate saccades toward the stimuli in the second paradigm were counted as errors and percentage errors were calculated to obtain a distractibility score. Twenty trials of the first and forty of the second paradigm were carried out to obtain saccadic latency and distractibility measures in each subject. Results revealed that all the participants had similar saccadic latencies; however, in comparison to both non-TD patients and normal controls, TD patients had a significantly higher distractibility score.

On the basis of these results we propose that TD-associated disruption of the nigrotectal pathway produces a subtle but distinct deficit in the control of saccadic system that manifests as increased distractibility. However, an abnormality in areas other than basal ganglia, such as frontal lobe, can also explain this finding of increased saccadic distractibility in TD patients. Other projections to the deeper layers of SC, for example, from the frontal eye fields may also play a similar inhibitory role.

CONCLUSION

We have reviewed preclinical evidence that suggests that GABAergic efferents from SNR play a critical role in mediation of basal ganglia function. Disruption of the efferents produces abnormal motor behavior including stereotypic and hyperkinetic involuntary movements in animals. Chronic neuroleptic treatment affects this GABA neuronal system and the changes are dyskinesia specific in primates. CSF GABA is found to be decreased in schizophrenic patients with TD compared to schizophrenic patients without TD. Control of the saccadic system, which is thought to be mediated by GABAergic efferents from SNR, is also found to be abnormal in schizophrenic patients with TD. Various studies have found that pharmacologic augmentation of brain GABA activity reduces dyskinetic symptoms in TD patients. On the basis of these clinical and preclinical evidences, we have hypothesized that in addition to the supersensitivity of DA receptors, hypofunction of nigral GABA activity plays a determinant role in the pathophysiology of TD.

REFERENCES

1. Klawans HL, Goetz CG, Perlik S: Tardive dyskinesia: review and update. Am J Psychiatry 137:900–906, 1980

2. Tarsy D, Baldessarini R: The pathophysiologic basis of tardive dyskinesia. Biol Psychiatry 12:431–450, 1977

3. Rupniak MN, Jenner P, Marsden CD: The effect of chronic neuroleptic administration on cerebral dopamine receptor function. Life Sci 32:2289–2311, 1985

4. MacKay AVP, Iversen, LL, Rosser M, et al: Increased brain dopamine and dopamine receptors in schizophrenia. Arch Gen Psychiatry 39:991–997, 1982

5. Gunne LM, Haggstrom JE, Sjoqust B: Association with persistent neuroleptic-induced dyskinesia or regional changes in brain GABA synthesis. Nature 309:347–349, 1984

6. Scheel-Kruger J: GABA. An eventual moderator and mediator in the basal ganglia system of dopamine related functions. Acta Neurol Scand 65 (Suppl 90):40–45, 1982

7. Gale K, Casu M: Dynamic utilization of GABA in substantia nigra: regulation by dopamine and GABA in the striatum, and its clinical and behavioral implications. Mol Cell Biochem 39:369–405, 1981

8. Beckstead RM, Frankfurter A: The distribution and some morphological features of substantia nigra neurons that project to the thalamus, superior colliculus and pedunculopontine nucleus in the monkey. Neuroscience 7:2377–2388, 1982

9. Hattori T, McCreer PL, Fibiger HC, et al: On the source of GABA-containing terminals in the substantia nigra: electron microscopic autoradiographic and biochemical studies. Brain Res 54:103–114, 1973

10. Oertel WH, Mugnaini E: Immunocytochemical studies of GABA-ergic neurons in rat basal ganglia and their relations to other neuronal system. Neurosci Lett 47:233–238, 1984

11. Muller P, Seeman P: Brain neurotransmitter receptors after long-term haloperidol: dopamine, acetylcholine, serotonin, alpha-noradrenergic and naloxone receptors. Life Sci 21:1751–1758, 1977

12. Smith RC, Davis JM: Behavioral supersensitivity to apomorphine and amphetamine after chronic high dose haloperidol treatment. Psychopharmacol Commun 1:285–293, 1975

13. Klawans HL, Rubovits R: An experimental model of tardive dyskinesia. J Neural Transm 33:235–246, 1972

14. Smith RC, Tamminga CA, Haraszti J, et al: Effects of dopamine agonists in tardive dyskinesia. Am J Psychiatry 134:763–768, 1977

15. Gerlach J, Reisby N, Randrup A: Dopaminergic hypersensitivity and cholinergic hypofunction in the pathophysiology of tardive dyskinesia. Psychopharmacologia 34:21–35, 1974

16. Fahn S: Long-term treatment of tardive dyskinesia with presynaptically acting dopamine-depleting agents, in Experimental Therapeutics of Movement Disorders. Edited by Fahn S, Calne DB, Shoalson I. New York, Raven Press, 1983, pp. 267–276

17. Smith R, Tamminga C, Chang J, et al: Dopaminergic agonist and antagonists in tardive dyskinesia. Am J Psychiatry 134:761–768, 1977

18. Pind K, Faurbye K: Concentration of homovanillic acid and 5-hydroxyindoleacetic acid in the cerebrospinal fluid after treatment with probenecid in patients with drug-induced tardive dyskinesia. Acta Psychiatr Scand 46:323–326, 1970

19. Riedever P, Jellinger K, Gabriel E: ^{3}H-spiperone binding to postmortem human putamen in paranoid and non-paranoid schizophrenics, in Psychiatry: The State of the Art. Edited by Pichot P. New York, Plenum Press, 1983, pp. 563–570

20. Crow TJ, Cross AJ, Johnstone EC, et al: Abnormal involuntary movements in schizophrenia: are they related to the disease process or its treatment? Are they associated with changes in dopamine receptors? J Clin Psychopharmacology 2:336–340, 1982

21. Tamminga CA, Smith RC, Pandey G, et al: A neuroendocrine study of supersensitivity in tardive dyskinesia. Arch Gen Psychiatry 34:1199–1203, 1977

22. Roberts E: A hypothesis suggesting that there is defect in the GABA system in schizophrenia. Neurosci Res Prog Bull 10:468–482, 1972

23. Anden NE, Stock G: Inhibiting effect of gamma-hydroxybutyric acid and gamma-aminobutyric acid on the dopamine cells in the substantia nigra. Naunyn Schmiedebergs Arch Pharmacol 279:89–92, 1973

24. Walters J, Lakoski J: Effect of muscimol on single unit activity of substantia nigra dopamine neurons. Eur J Pharmacol 47:469–471, 1978

25. Domesick VB: The anatomical basis for feedback and feedforward in the striatonigral system, in Apomorphine and Other Dopaminomimetics (Volume 1). Edited by Gessa GL, Corsini GU. New York, Raven Press, 1981, pp. 27–39

26. Kilpatrick IC, Collingridge GL, Starr MS: Evidence for the participation of nigrotectal gamma-aminobutyrate containing neurons in striatal and nigral-derived circling in the rat. Neuroscience 7:207–222, 1982

27. Di Chiara G, Morselli M, Porceddu ML, et al: Evidence that nigral GABA mediates behavioral responses elicited by striatal dopamine receptor stimulation. Life Sci 23:2045–2052, 1978

28. Childs JA, Gale K: Evidence that the nigrotegmental GABAergic projection mediates stereotypy induced by apomorphine and intranigral muscimol. Life Sci 33:1007–1010, 1983

29. Cools AK, Jaspers R, Kolasiewicz W, et al: Substantia nigra as a station that not only transmits, but also transforms incoming signals for its behavioral expression: striatal dopamine and GABA-mediated responses of pars reticulata neurons. Behav Brain Res 7:39–49, 1983

30. Scheel-Kruger J, Arnt J, Magelund G: Behavioral stimulation induced by muscimol and other GABA agonists injected into the substantia nigra. Neurosci Lett 4:351–356, 1977

31. Papadopoulos G, Houston JP: Removal of the telencephalon spaces turning induced by injection of GABA agonists and antagonists into the substantia nigra. Behav Brain Res 1:25–38, 1980

32. Gale K, Mariano C: Functional regulation of GABA turnover and GABA receptors in the nigrostriatal system: interaction with dopamine, in GABA and Basal Ganglia. Edited by Dichiara G, Gessa GL. New York, Raven Press, 1981, pp. 86–93

33. Reavill C, Leigh N, Jenner P, et al: GABA mediated circling from substantia nigra [letter]. Nature 287:368, 1980

34. Mao CC, Cheney DL, Marco E, et al: Turnover times of gamma-aminobutyric acid and acetylcholine in nucleus caudatus, nucleus accumbens, globus pallidus, and substantia nigra: effects of repeated administration of haloperidol. Brain Res 132:375–379, 1977

35. Gunne LM, Haggstrom JE: Reductions of nigral glutamic acid decarboxylase in rats with neuroleptic-induced oral dyskinesia. Psychopharmacology 81:191–194, 1983

36. Itoh M: Effect of haloperidol on glutamate decarboxylase activity in discrete brain areas of the rat. Psychopharmacology 79:169–172, 1983

37. Gale K: Chronic blockade of dopamine receptors by antischizophrenic drugs enhances GABA binding in substantia nigra. Nature 283:569–570, 1980

38. Freed WJ, Gillin JC, Wyatt RJ: Anomalous behavioral response to imidazoleacetic acid, a GABA agonist, in animals treated chronically with haloperidol. Biol Psychiatry 15:21–35, 1980

39. Warczak BL, Hume C, Walters JR: Supersensitivity of substantia nigra pars reticulata neurons to GABAergic drugs after striatal lesions. Life Sci 28:2411–2420, 1981

40. Waddington JL, Cross AJ: Denervation supersensitivity in the striatonigral GABA pathway. Nature 276:618–620, 1978

41. Saji M, Reis DJ: Delayed transneuronal death of substantia nigra neurons prevented by gamma aminobutyric acid agonist. Science 235:66–69, 1987

42. Olianas MC, DeMontis GM, Concu A, et al: Intranigral kainic acid: evidence for nigral non-dopaminergic neurons controlling posture and behaviour in a manner opposite to the dopaminergic ones. Eur J Pharmacol 49:223–232, 1978

43. Olianas MC, DeMontis GM, Mulas G, et al: The striatal dopaminergic function is mediated by the inhibition of a nigral, non-dopaminergic neuronal system via a striato-nigral GABAergic pathway. Eur J Pharmacol 49:233–241, 1978b

44. Hikosaka O, Wurtz RH: Modification of saccadic eye movements by GABA-related substances I: Effects of muscimol in monkey substantia nigra pars reticulata. J Neurophysiol 53:266–291, 1985

45. Hikosaka O, Wurtz RH: Modification of saccadic eye movements by GABA-related substances II: Effects of muscimol in monkey substantia nigra pars reticulata. J Neurophysiol 53:292–308, 1985

46. Casu M, Gale K: Effects of gamma-vinyl-GABA on dopamine neurons: relationship between elevation of GABA in nerve-terminals and change in tyrosine hydroxylase activity. Fed Proc 4:290, 1981

47. Enna SJ (ed): The GABA Receptors. Clifton, NJ, Humana Press, 1983

48. Enna SJ: GABA receptors, in The Gaba Receptors. Edited by Enna SJ. Clifton, NJ, Humana Press, 1983, pp. 1–18

49. Bowery NG, Hill DR, Hudson AL, et al: Baclofen decreases neurotransmitter release in the mammalian CNS by an action at a novel GABA receptor. Nature 283:92–94, 1980

50. Tamminga CA, Crayton J, Chase T: Improvement in tardive dyskinesia after muscimol therapy. Arch Gen Psychiatry 36:595–598, 1979

51. Korsgaard S, Casey D, Gerlach J, et al: The effect of tetrahydroisoxazolopyridinol (THIP) in tardive dyskinesia. Arch Gen Psychiatry 39:1017–1021, 1982

52. Thaker GK, Tamminga CA, Alphs, LD, et al: Brain GABA abnormality in tardive dyskinesia. Arch Gen Psychiatry 44:522–529, 1987

53. Hosli E, Korsgaard-Larsen P, Hosli L: Autoradiographic localization of binding sites for the gamma-aminobutyric acid analogues 4,5,6,7-tetra-hydroisoxazolo [5,4-c] pyridine-3-ol (THIP), isoguvacine and baclofen on cultured neurons of rat cerebellum and spinal cord. Neurosci Lett 61:153–157, 1985

54. Sevestre P, Roudot P, Bathieu N, et al: The effect of progabide, a specific GABA-ergic agonist, on neuroleptic-induced tardive dyskinesia: results of a pilot study. Presented at 13th Collegium Internationale Neuropsychopharmacologicum, Jerusalem, 1982

55. Morselli PL, Bossi L, Henry JF, et al: On the therapeutic action of SL 76 002, a new GABA-neurotransmission. Brain Res Bull 5(Suppl 2):411–414, 1980

56. Thaker GK, Hare TA, Tamminga CA: GABA neuronal hypofunction in neuroleptic-induced dyskinesias. Presented at 15th Collegium Internationale Psychopharmalogicum Meeting, Puerto Rico, 1986

57. Loscher W: GABA in plasma and cerebrospinal fluid of different species. Effects of gamma-acetylenic GABA, gamma-vinyl GABA and sodium valproate. J Neurochem 32:1587–1591, 1979

58. Jung M, Lippert B, Metcalf B, et al: Gamma-vinyl GABA (4-amino-hex-5-enoic acid), a new selective irreversible inhibitor of GABA-T: effects on brain GABA metabolism in mice. J Neurochem 29:797–802, 1977

59. Grove J, Schechter P, Tell G, et al: Increased gamma-aminobutyric acid (GABA), homocarnosine and B-alanine in cerebrospinal fluid of patients treated without vinyl GABA. Life Sci 28:2431–2439, 1981

60. Hammond EJ, Wilder BJ: Gamma-vinyl GABA: a new antiepileptic drug. Clin Neuropharmacol 8:1–12, 1985

61. Casey D, Gerlach J, Magelund G, et al: Gamma-acetylenic GABA in tardive dyskinesia. Arch Gen Psychiatry 37:1376–1379, 1980

62. Tell GP, Schechter PJ, Koch-Weser J, et al: Effects of gamma-vinyl GABA. N Engl J Med 305:581–582, 1981

63. Tamminga CA, Thaker GK, Hare T, et al: GABA agonist therapy improves tardive dyskinesia. Lancet 2:97–98, 1983

64. Korsgaard S, Casey DE, Gerlach J: Effect of gamma-vinyl GABA in tardive dyskinesia. Psychiatry Res 8:261–269, 1983

65. Haefely W: Benzodiazepine interactions with GABA receptors. Neurosci Lett 47:201–206, 1984

66. Ticku MK: Benzodiazepine GABA receptor-ionophore complex. Neuropharmacology 22:1459–1470, 1983

67. Skerritt JH, McDonald RL: Benzodiazepine receptor ligand actions on GABA responses, B-carbolines, purines. Eur J Pharmacol 101:135–141, 1984

68. Singh MM, Becker RE, Pitman RK, et al: Diazepam-induced changes in tardive dyskinesia: suggestions for a new conceptual model. Biol Psychiatry 17:729–742, 1982

69. Saito T, Ishizawa H, Tsuchiya F, et al: Neurochemical findings in the cerebrospinal fluid of schizophrenic patients with tardive dyskinesia and neuroleptic-induced parkinsonism. Jpn J Psychiatr Neurol 40:189–194, 1986

70. Hare TA: Alterations of central GABAergic activity in neurological and psychiatric disorders: evaluation through measurements of GABA and GAD activity in cerebrospinal fluid. Mol Cell Biochem 39:297–304, 1981

71. Kuriyama K, Sze PY: Blood–brain barrier to ^{3}H-gamma-aminobutyric acid in normal and aminooxyacetic acid-treated animals. Neuropharmacology 10:103–108, 1971

72. Wood JH, Hare TA, Enna SL, et al: Sites of origin and rostrocaudal concentration gradients of GABA in cerebrospinal fluid. Brain Res Bull 5(Suppl 2):111–114, 1980

73. Manyam NVB, Hare TA, Katz L: Effects of isoniazid on cerebrospinal fluid and plasma GABA levels in Huntington's disease. Life Sci 26:1303–1308, 1980

74. Grossman MH, Hare TA, Manyam NVB: Stability of GABA levels in CSF under various conditions of storage. Brain Res 182:99–106, 1980

75. Ferraro TN, Hare TA: Triple-column ion-exchange physiological amino acid analysis with fluorescent detection: baseline characterization of human cerebrospinal fluid. Ann Biochem 143:82–94, 1984

76. Thaker GK, Nguyen JA, Ferraro TM, et al: Neuronal hypofunction in tardive dyskinesia: CSF GABA levels and saccadic eye movements. Society of Neurosciences Abstract 12:479, 1986

Chapter 15

Calcium Channel Antagonists: Interaction with Dopamine, Schizophrenia, and Tardive Dyskinesia

Richard L. Borison, M.D., Ph.D.
Michael C. McLarnon, M.D.
Nicholas DeMartines, M.D.
Bruce I. Diamond, Ph.D.

Chapter 15

Calcium Channel Antagonists: Interaction with Dopamine, Schizophrenia, and Tardive Dyskinesia

Voltage-dependent calcium (Ca^{++}) channels that mediate functions of smooth muscle, cardiac muscle, and neural tissue are blocked by Ca^{++} channel antagonist drugs (1, 2). Ca^{++} channel blockers can be divided into the dihydropyridines (for example, nifedipine), papaverine derivatives (verapamil), piperazine derivatives (fluparazine), and benzothiazepines (diltiazem). Receptor sites for the dihydropyridine class of Ca^{++} channel antagonists can be labeled with ligands such as ^{3}H-nitrendipine (3). In contrast, Ca^{++} channel blockers of the verapamil and diltiazem class do not interact at the dihydropyridine site but act at a distinct site that is allosterically linked to the ^{3}H-nitrendipine sites (4). Recent studies suggest that dihydropyridine binding sites in brain correspond to Ca^{++} channel function (5), and Ca^{++} channel binding sites are concentrated in the limbic and extrapyramidal system as well as cortex.

There appears to be a role for Ca^{++} channel blockers in dopamine (DA) function, as demonstrated by verapamil's inhibiting DA release from the arcuate nucleus (6), their benefit in the treatment of movement disorders (7), the direct competition with DA for dopamine-2 (D-2) receptor binding in the striatum (8), and their apparent therapeutic benefit in mania (9), temporal lobe epilepsy (10), and schizophrenia (11). Moreover, certain neuroleptics that block DA receptors also act as Ca^{++} channel blockers (12). These DA blocking drugs include the diphenylbutylpiperidines (for example, pimozide, penfluridol), which are structurally similar to verapamil. Thioridazine and clozapine also possess relatively potent Ca^{++} channel blocking activities. The occurrence of fewer extrapyramidal side effects (7), lack of prolactin release (13), and the response of not only positive but negative symptoms of schizophrenia (12) observed with some of these neuroleptics, compared to neuroleptics without significant Ca^{++} channel inhibition, argue for the possible benefits of concomitant blockade of Ca^{++} channels and D-2 receptors in the treatment of certain neuropsychiatric disorders.

Since both clinical and biochemical evidence point to the beneficial action of drugs that possess Ca^{++} channel and DA receptor blocking properties, as well as the actions of Ca^{++} channel blockage alone on DA function, we have conducted clinical and animal studies directed at the functional in vivo effects of these interactions.

ANIMAL STUDIES

Method

All procedures in animals were performed on male Sprague-Dawley rats (200 to 250 g). We studied the effects of Ca^{++} channel entry blockers on 1) DA-agonist (apomorphine or amphetamine)-induced-stereotypy, 2) DA-agonist-induced rotations in animals with unilateral 6-hydroxydopamine lesions of the substantia nigra, 3) neuroleptic (chlorpromazine)-induced striatal DA receptor supersensitivity, and 4) DA receptor binding (^{3}H-spiroperidol) in the striatum. The action of Ca^{++} blockers injected directly into rat striatum during DA-agonist-induced stereotypy was also studied.

Results

Diltiazem and nifedipine, even at high doses, had no effect on apomorphine-induced stereotypy alone or in combination with chlorpromazine. Verapamil, only at high doses (50 mg/kg), when coadministered with chlorpromazine, significantly potentiated ($p < 0.05$) chlorpromazine antagonism of amphetamine-induced stereotypy. Verapamil when given alone also showed significant antagonism to amphetamine-induced stereotypy, but this was not demonstrated in a clear dose–response relationship. In contrast, low doses of nifedipine and verapamil potentiated amphetamine stereotypy at 90 and 120 minutes after injection. In substantia-nigra-lesioned animals, verapamil (50 mg/kg) significantly antagonized both apomorphine- and amphetamine-induced rotations, but not at lower dosages. In contrast, diltiazem potentiated amphetamine ipsilateral rotations while not affecting apomorphine contralateral turning, and nifedipine had no significant effect on either of the DA-agonist-induced rotations.

The administration of verapamil or diltiazem to the caudate nucleus did not produce any behavioral response per se. Verapamil in doses of 1 to 10 $\mu g/\mu l$ when locally applied to the striatum inhibited the systemic effects of both apomorphine and amphetamine stereotypy, which was significant at the $p < 0.05$ level. None of the other Ca^{++} channel blockers affected the stereotyped behavior induced by either of the DA agonists.

In the tardive dyskinesia animal model, the 21-day administration of chlorpromazine led to behavioral striatal supersensitivity as measured by the enhanced behavioral response of these animals to apomorphine compared to saline controls. Of the three Ca^{++} channel blockers, only verapamil produced any effects. Chronic treatment with verapamil alone resulted in DA striatal subsensitivity to apomorphine treatment. Although the addition of verapamil to chlorpromazine for 21 days led to an antagonism of striatal supersensitivity, this effect did not reach statistical significance. None of the Ca^{++} blocking drugs affected neuroleptic-induced supersensitivity markedly.

Inhibition of in vitro spiroperidol binding in the striatum was observed only with verapamil and not other Ca^{++} channel blockers. The inhibition of spiroperidol receptor binding by verapamil occurred at a concentration of $1 \times 10\text{-}6M$.

CLINICAL STUDY

Method

The subjects in the study were 13 chronic male schizophrenic patients who had signed informed consent to participate in the project. The average age of the subjects was 43.4 years (SD = ± 6.3 years), and they had been continuously hospitalized for a mean of 7.4 years (SD = ± 3.2 years). These subjects were considered treatment refractory patients as defined by failing to have had a good response to antipsychotic medication during the previous 5 years, during which time they had been treated with a minimum of three neuroleptic agents from at least two different structural classes, in doses that were minimally equivalent to 1000 mg of chlorpromazine.

All subjects were placed on 600 mg chlorpromazine for a minimum of 2 weeks to allow for stabilization of psychopathology, and were then begun on verapamil treatment, 240 mg daily, in three divided doses. The dosing regimen was flexible, with a maximum dose of 480 mg in three divided doses. During the 2-week baseline period, and during the 6 weeks of joint verapamil–chlorpromazine therapy, weekly assessments of psychopathology were performed using the Brief Psychiatric Rating Scale (BPRS) (14) and the Scale for Assessment of Negative Symptoms (SANS) (15). Neurological side effects were determined using the Abnormal Involuntary Movement Scale (AIMS) (16). At the end of verapamil treatment, an additional rating was performed 1 week after verapamil treatment while subjects were still maintained on 600 mg chlorpromazine.

Results

In general, the combination of verapamil plus chlorpromazine was well tolerated, the only important side effect occurring being orthostatic hypotension. This side effect occurred primarily in the morning before patients had become physically active and resulted in an occasional dose of medication being held. Patients were largely asymptomatic, and no syncopal episodes occurred. Patients reached maximal doses of verapamil (480 mg/day) by the third week of treatment.

The effects of combining verapamil with chlorpromazine were

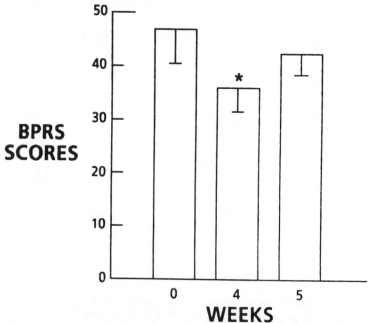

Figure 1. The effects of joint administration of verapamil and chlorpromazine on psychosis as measured by the Brief Psychiatric Rating Scale (BPRS). At week 0, only chlorpromazine was administered, but by week 4 of additional treatment with verapamil, there was a statistically significant decrease in BPRS scores. At the beginning of week 5 verapamil was discontinued, and BPRS scores increased to their baseline values.* p < 0.05.

significant on the BPRS. As shown in Figure 1, the addition of verapamil produced a significant ($p < 0.05$) decrease in BPRS scores that was maximal at the fourth week of joint treatment, whereas BPRS scores returned to baseline levels at 1 week after verapamil treatment. An analysis of BPRS items showed the greatest effect on emotional withdrawal, with a significant reduction ($p < 0.05$) in severity of this symptom. Likewise, analysis of SANS scores (Figure 2) revealed a similar reduction in the severity of negative symptoms ($p < 0.05$) that was maximal by the third week of treatment and reversed itself after verapamil was terminated.

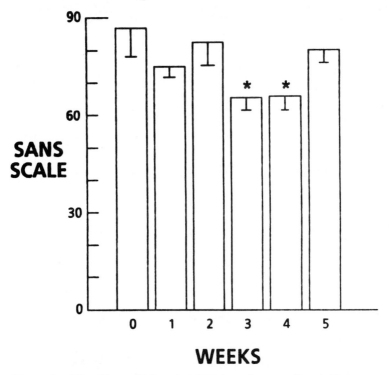

Figure 2.   The effects of joint administration of verapamil and chlorpromazine on psychosis as measured by the Scale for Assessment of Negative Symptoms (SANS). At week 0, only chlorpromazine was administered, whereas verapamil treatment was initiated during week 1. By weeks 3 and 4, there was a significant decrease in negative symptomatology. At the beginning of week 5 verapamil was discontinued, and SANS scores increased to their baseline values.* $p < 0.05$.

The majority of patients had a preexisting tardive dyskinesia, averaging 12.75 (SD = ± 3.7) on AIMS testing. The addition of verapamil produced a dramatic lowering of AIMS scores ($p < 0.01$) in nearly every patient, reaching greatest therapeutic benefit by the third week of treatment and approaching baseline levels when verapamil was discontinued (Figure 3).

DISCUSSION

There are two basic mechanisms by which calcium is made accessible to the intracellular space. One mechanism involves the release of Ca^{++} by the endoplasmic reticulum. This effect is triggered by cell receptor mechanisms that stimulate the metabolism of phosphatidylinositol biphosphate to diacylglycerol and inositol triphosphate

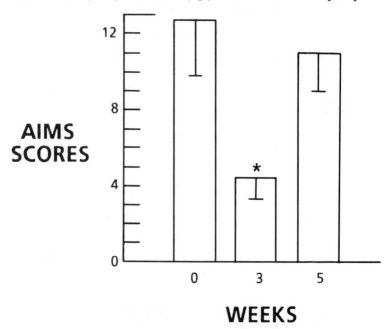

Figure 3. The effects of joint administration of verapamil and chlorpromazine on tardive dyskinesia as measured by the Abnormal Involuntary Movement Scale (AIMS). At week 0, only chlorpromazine was administered, but by week 3 of additional treatment with verapamil, there was a maximal level of suppression of dyskinesias. At the beginning of week 5 verapamil was discontinued, and AIMS scores increased to their baseline values.
* $p < 0.01$.

(17). The second major mechanism is when the cell membrane changes its permeability to Ca^{++} allowing this ion to move along its electrochemical gradient from the extracellular to intracellular space. This latter mechanism may also be regulated by receptor mechanisms, but seems particularly dependent on cell membrane voltage, and hence are termed voltage-sensitive Ca^{++} channels. The influx of Ca^{++} into the neuron has various actions, including changes in cell excitability, the release of neurotransmitters, and the activation of Ca^{++}-dependent enzymes, including calmodulin-dependent protein kinase, as well as other kinases (1).

The voltage-sensitive Ca^{++} channels contain specific receptors for the dihydropyridines, with receptors for other Ca^{++} channel antagonists (for example, verapamil, diltiazem) appearing to have an allosteric interaction with the dihydropyridine binding site. The physiological actions of these receptors are still being investigated (18), since there appear to be multiple calcium channels present in nervous tissue, all of which differ in their physiological functions. It has been hypothesized that the dihydropyridine binding site may not be linked with neurotransmitter release (19).

DA-agonist-induced stereotyped behavior in animals is mediated via striatal D-2 receptor mechanisms. The ability of drugs to block this behavior is used to determine antipsychotic drug activity and DA receptor antagonism. The actions of chlorpromazine in antagonizing DA agonist stereotypy is consistent with this hypothesis. The failure of moderate doses (10 to 25 mg/kg) of diltiazem and nifedipine to antagonize apomorphine stereotypy when given alone or concomitantly with chlorpromazine suggests a lack of centrally mediated DA antagonist effects for these agents. In contrast, high doses of verapamil (50 mg/kg) antagonized amphetamine stereotypy when administered in combination with chlorpromazine. Thus, it would appear that only this Ca^{++} channel antagonist possesses DA receptor antagonist properties.

Similar to the blockade of DA-agonist-induced stereotypy, blockage of D-2 receptors in the caudate nucleus antagonizes ipsilateral and contralateral rotations produced by amphetamine and apomorphine in animals with unilateral lesions of the substantia nigra. In this model, only high doses of verapamil antagonized rotations, thereby exhibiting anti-DA effects. As with DA-mediated stereotyped behavior, nifedipine and diltiazem lacked DA blocking properties. Unexpectedly, diltiazem potentiated amphetamine turning, which could be the result of enhanced DA presynaptic release via either Ca^{++} channel effects or blockade of presynaptic DA autoreceptors.

The local application of Ca^{++} channel antagonists to the striatum did not produce any behavioral effects. With the exception of verapamil, local applications of these drugs to the striatum did not affect behaviors produced by systemic DA agonist treatment. Again verapamil was the only Ca^{++} channel antagonist to exert an antagonistic effect, thereby indicating some actions on DA receptor blockade. In agreement with this hypothesis were the results that only verapamil inhibited in vitro spiroperidol receptor binding. The inhibition of DA receptor binding and DA stereotypy by verapamil occurred in the mM range.

The question as to whether the lack of DA receptor effects observed with the other Ca^{++} channel blockers is due to their inability to cross the blood–brain barrier can be refuted by the absence of their effects when injected directly into the brain. Moreover, our results suggest that large amounts of verapamil are required (50 mg/kg) to achieve brain DA blockade (mM). This may be due to either a poor penetration of the blood–brain barrier or a relatively nonspecific action at dopaminergic sites.

Verapamil is a lipid-soluble compound and of all the commercially available Ca^{++} channel blockers at this time is probably the best candidate for penetrating the blood–brain barrier. This prediction appears to be corroborated by the ability to measure verapamil and its metabolite in the cerebrospinal fluid of patients receiving this medication (20, 21).

There are, at this point, limited clinical data concerning the effects of Ca^{++} channel blockers in psychiatric illness. Dubovsky et al. first reported the efficacy of verapamil in a manic patient (22) and in two subsequent reports have studied the efficacy of verapamil in 10 additional manic patients using a placebo cross-over design (23). They found verapamil to be helpful in eight patients, with the antimanic effect reaching clinical significance. In two separate reports (9, 24), Giannini et al. reported on the actions of verapamil in 30 manic patients. They observed that verapamil was equally efficacious with lithium and superior to clonidine treatment. In the several studies in which Ca^{++} channel blockers were combined with neuroleptic or lithium treatment (17, 25, 26, 28), 19 of 22 patients who were diagnosed as manic or schizoaffective showed definite improvement with this combination therapy. The reports of verapamil's actions in depression are even more limited; however, one case report (29) and one report (open study) on 19 depressives indicated a therapeutic action for verapamil (25). The doses of verapamil used were between 160 and 480 mg daily in these studies of affective disorders.

The calcium channel blockers are believed to affect the interaction of calcium and calmodulin. This coupling is necessary for the activation of second messengers and neurotransmitter release (30). Not only has it previously been noted that neuroleptics interact with calmodulin, but it is also suggested that the more potent calcium-channel-blocking neuroleptics may putatively have a greater effect in reversing the negative symptoms of schizophrenia (12). If this is true, it would then seem logical that potentiating the calcium-channel-blocking activity of a neuroleptic, by the addition of verapamil, may increase the efficacy of a neuroleptic in the treatment of chronic negative-symptom schizophrenic patients.

It is of theoretical interest that those neuroleptic drugs which are both DA receptor and Ca^{++} channel blockers appear to produce less DA-mediated central side-effects, for example, thioridazine, clozapine, and pimozide. It has been argued that the relative lack of DA-induced striatal supersensitivity in animals and neurological side effects in humans produced by drugs such as clozapine was due to these drugs' greater intrinsic anticholinergic activity. This viewpoint, however, has not been experimentally or clinically substantiated, and other mechanisms must be investigated (31).

In studying the ability of chronic pimozide to produce a decrease in the number of striatal D-2 receptors compared to the increase observed with haloperidol (32), it has been argued that this may be the result of the concomitant DA receptor and Ca^{++} channel antagonism produced by pimozide. Another neuroleptic with this dual property, clozapine (7), rarely produces tardive dyskinesia. In our animal studies with chronic verapamil and chlorpromazine, the expected supersensitive striatal response to DA agonists was observed in chlorpromazine-treated animals. In contrast, concomitant verapamil did not markedly affect this supersensitivity, but when given alone it did produce a subsensitivity response. In contrast, it has been demonstrated that the receptor proliferation induced by neuroleptic treatment in animals can be reversed by Ca^{++} channel blockers (33). Thus the effect of pimozide in decreasing striatal DA receptor number may be explained as involving its Ca^{++} antagonist properties. Furthermore, this may also explain the palliative effect of verapamil on tardive dyskinesia that was observed in our study population.

Since all neuroleptics are effective in ameliorating the positive symptoms of schizophrenia, the involvement of D-2 receptors in the manifestation of these symptoms seems apparent (12). Since pimozide has been reported to be effective not only on positive symptoms, but also on negative symptoms of schizophrenia, the Ca^{++} channel antagonist property of pimozide has been evoked to explain its unique action on negative symptomatology. Thus, Ca^{++} channel antagonism alone may be required to treat negative symptoms, or the combination of DA receptor and Ca^{++} channel blockade may be required. In one of the few well-controlled studies of calcium channel blockers in psychiatric illness, Pickar et al. (21) administered verapamil using a placebo-controlled double-blind design to seven otherwise drug-free schizophrenic subjects. They failed to find a therapeutic effect, but rather observed a worsening of hostility and uncooperativeness in patients. These changes in mental status were correlated with verapamil producing an increase in serum prolactin levels and an increase in plasma and CSF levels of homovanillic acid. In another double-blind placebo-controlled study involving the addition of verapamil to either haloperidol or loxitane treatment in schizophrenic subjects (34), it was observed that there were no statistical differences between verapamil and placebo treatments. Also of interest are the reports that verapamil has proved effective in treating individual cases of Tourette's syndrome and tardive dyskinesia (35–37).

The inconsistency in results in treating schizophrenia with calcium channel blockers may be explained in several different ways. In our study, patients were older and had more chronic courses than in the other studies. Furthermore, negative signs played a significant role in the clinical picture of our subject population. Perhaps if Ca^{++} channel blockers play an important role in ameliorating negative signs, this may explain the therapeutic benefit observed in our study. However, our data need to be corroborated in double-blind placebo-controlled studies and at this time can only be considered highly suggestive for a therapeutic role for Ca^{++} channel blockers in schizophrenia. Furthermore, the small numbers of patients treated in these studies make it impossible to generalize on the lack or presence of therapeutic benefit of verapamil in schizophrenia.

It would appear that the Ca^{++} channel blockers offer a possible alternative treatment strategy in mania or schizophrenia when other treatment modalities have failed. Furthermore, the possible role for these drugs in ameliorating tardive dyskinesia may hold great promise.

REFERENCES

1. Godfrain T, Miller R, Wibo M: Calcium antagonism and calcium entry blockade. Pharmacol Rev 38:321–416, 1986

2. Fleckenstein A: Specific pharmacology of calcium in myocardium, cardiac pacemakers, and vascular smooth muscle. Annu Rev Pharmacol Toxicol 17:149–166, 1977

3. Gould RJ, Murphy KMM, Snyder SH: [³H]Nitrendipine-labeled calcium channels discriminate inorganic calcium agonists and antagonists. Proc Natl Acad Sci USA 79:3656–3660, 1982

4. Murphy KMM, Gould RJ, Largent BL, et al: A unitary mechanism of calcium antagonism drug action. Proc Natl Acad Sci USA 80:860–864, 1983

5. Middlemiss DN, Spedding M: A functional correlate for the dihydropyridine binding site in rat brain. Nature 314:94–96, 1985

6. Ehlert FJ, Roeske WR, Itoga E, et al: The binding of [³H]nitrendipine to receptors for calcium antagonists in the heart, cerebral cortex and ileum of rats. Life Sci 30:2191–2204, 1982

7. DiRenzo G, Amoroso S, Taglialatela M, et al: Dual effects of verapamil on K-evoked release of endogenous dopamine from arcuate nucleus–median eminence complex. Neurosci Lett 50:269-272

8. Goldstein JA: Calcium and neurotransmission. Biol Psychiatry 19:465–466, 1984

9. DeVries DJ, Beart PM: Competitive inhibition of [³H]spiroperidol binding to D-2 dopamine receptors in striatal homogenates by organic calcium channel antagonists and polyvalent cations. Eur J Pharmacol 106:133–139, 1985

10. Giannini AJ, Houser WL, Lorselle RH, et al: Antimanic effects of verapamil. Am J Psychiatry 141:1602–1603, 1984

11. Overweg J, Binnie CD, Meijer JWA, et al: Double blind placebo controlled trial of flunarizine as add-on therapy in epilepsy. Epilepsia 25:217–222, 1984

12. Giannini AJ, Loiselle R: Calcium channel blockers and psychopathology (Abstract No. 612.10). Presented at the Fourth World Congress on Biological Psychiatry, Philadelphia, PA, 1985

13. Gould RJ, Murphy KMM, Reynolds IJ, et al: Antischizophrenic drugs of the diphenylbutylpiperidine type act as calcium channel antagonists. Proc Natl Acad Sci USA 80:5122–5125, 1983

14. Denef C, Van Mueten JM, Leysen JE, et al: Evidence that pimozide is not a partial agonist of dopamine receptors. Life Sci 25:217–226, 1979

15. Overall JE, Gorham DR: The brief psychiatric rating scale (BPRS). Psychol Rep 10:799–812, 1962

16. Andreasen NC: Negative symptoms in schizophrenia. Arch Gen Psychiatry 39:784–790, 1982

17. Guy W: ECDEU Assessment Manual for Psychopharmacology. Washington, DC, U.S. Department of Health, Education and Welfare, 1976

18. Abdel-Latif AA: Calcium-mobilizing receptors, polyphosphoinositides, and the generation of second messengers. Pharmacol Rev 38:227–272, 1986

19. Greenberg DA: Calcium channels and calcium channel antagonists. Ann Neurol 21:317–330, 1987

20. Miller RJ: Multiple calcium channels and neuronal function. Science 235:46–52, 1987

21. Doran AR, Narang PK, Meigs CY, et al: Verapamil concentrations in cerebrospinal fluid after oral administration. N Engl J Med 312:1261–1262, 1985

22. Pickar D, Wolkowitz OM, Doran AR, et al: Clinical and biochemical effects of verapamil administration to schizophrenic patients. Arch Gen Psychiatry 44:113–118, 1987

23. Dubovsky SL, Franks RD, Lifscitz M: Effectiveness of verapamil in the treatment of a manic patient. Am J Psychiatry 139:502–504, 1982

24. Dubovsky SL: Calcium antagonists: a new class of psychiatric drugs? Psychiatric Annals 16:724–728, 1986

25. Giannini AJ, Loiselle RH, Price WA, et al: Comparison of antimanic efficacy of clonidine and verapamil. J Clin Pharmacol 25:307–308, 1985

26. Hoschl C, Blahos J, Kabes J: The use of calcium channel blockers in psychoses, in Biological Psychiatry 1985. Edited by Shagass CE, Josiasson RC, Bridger WH, et al. New York, Elsevier, 1986, pp. 330–332

27. Caillard V: Treatment of mania using a calcium channel antagonist—preliminary trial. Neuropsychobiology 14:23–26, 1985

28. Dose M, Emrich HM: Antimanic properties of verapamil, in Biological Psychiatry 1985. Edited by Shagass CE, Josiasson RC, Bridger WH, et al. New York, Elsevier, 1986, pp. 320–322

29. Brotman AW, Fahardi AM, Gelenberg AJ: Verapamil treatment in acute mania. J Clin Psychiatry 47:136–138, 1986

30. Hoschl C: Verapamil for depression? (Letter to editor). Am J Psychiatry 140:1100, 1983

31. DeLorenzo RJ: Calcium-calmodulin systems in psychopharmacology and synaptic modulation. Psychopharmacol Bull 19:393–397, 1983

32. Borison RL: Pharmacology of antipsychotic drugs. J Clin Psychiatry 46 (4, Section 2): 25–28, 1985

33. Tecott HL, Kwong LL, Uhr S: Differential modulation of dopamine D2 receptors by chronic haloperidol, nitrendipine, and pimozide. Biol Psychiatry 21:1114–1122, 1986

34. Grebb JA, Shelton RC, Freed WJ: Calcium blockers prevent dopamine hypersensitivity. Presented at annual meeting of the American Psychiatric Association, Washington, DC, 1986

35. Grebb JA, Shelton RC, Taylor EH, et al: A negative, double-blind, placebo controlled, clinical trial of verapamil in chronic schizophrenia. Biol Psychiatry 21:691–694, 1986

36. Goldstein JA: Nifedipine treatment of Tourette's syndrome. J Clin Psychiatry 45:360, 1984

37. Walsh TL, Lavenstein B, Licamele WL, et al: Calcium antagonists in the treatment of Tourette's disorder. Am J Psychiatry 143:1467–1468, 1986

38. Barlow N, Childs A: An anti-tardive-dyskinesia effect of verapamil. Am J Psychiatry 143:1485, 1986

Chapter 16

Treatment of the On-Off Dyskinesia Syndrome of Parkinson's Disease with New Drug Delivery Technologies for Selective Dopamine-2 Receptor Agonists

Stephen Michael Stahl, M.D., Ph.D.

Chapter 16

Treatment of the On-Off Dyskinesia Syndrome of Parkinson's Disease with New Drug Delivery Technologies for Selective Dopamine-2 Receptor Agonists

Studies of dyskinesias in Huntington's chorea contributed to the formulation of the dopamine theory of tardive dyskinesia (TD). Investigation of abnormal movements in other neurological disorders, such as the on–off dyskinesia syndrome of Parkinson's disease, may provide useful information for the understanding of the phenomenology of TD. The mainstay of the treatment of Parkinson's disease is levodopa, usually prescribed with a peripheral dopa decarboxylase inhibitor. In most patients the initial response to levodopa is excellent, but after several years problems begin to develop. Efficacy of levodopa seems to diminish and this can only temporarily be overcome by increasing the dose. The length of action of each dose gets shorter, and parkinsonian features return before the next dose is due (wearing-off effect). Dyskinesias (usually chorea) develop at the time of peak dose and these may extend throughout the whole period of benefit. As the response to each dose becomes shorter and more unpredictable, patients find themselves switching several times a day from a state of mobility with dyskinesias to one of profound parkinsonism. Such motor fluctuations are known as the "on–off syndrome"(1). For patients with onset of Parkinson's disease at a young age, having many years of levodopa therapy ahead of them, on–off fluctuations appear to be inevitable sooner or later.

The on–off syndrome as described above is one of the major problems associated with long-term levodopa therapy. It highlights the needs for additional antiparkinsonian therapy, such as dopamine agonists, for the prevention and treatment of motor fluctuations. Thus, two major treatment issues must be addressed.

First, there is evidence to suggest that deferring treatment with levodopa in the early stages of Parkinson's disease may prevent the subsequent development of motor fluctuations (2), although not all authorities agree with this (3). Early treatment with bromocriptine may postpone the need for levodopa therapy or may allow a lower dose to be prescribed (4). However, many patients develop side effects with higher doses of bromocriptine, and few derive enough benefit to manage without levodopa for long (5). In addition, bromocriptine, which has a complex chemical structure, is expensive to manufacture. There is a need for a highly potent, reasonably priced dopamine agonist that can be taken on a long-term basis without side effects.

Second, there is the problem of treating on–off fluctuations once they have developed. The fluctuations can be abolished with continuous intravenous infusions of levodopa, which seem to work by producing constant levodopa blood level (6–8). This avoids the peaks and troughs that occur with oral levodopa, even when small doses are taken frequently. Various attempts have been made to adapt the concept of continuous drug infusion for practical use. Oral slow-release levodopa preparations (Sinemet CR and Madopar HBS), dopa methylester infusions, and subcutaneous lisuride infusions have all been tried and have all had their problems (9–12). There is a need for a potent dopaminergic agent that can be delivered at a constant rate in a practical manner.

This chapter reviews the properties of a new selective dopamine-2 (D-2) receptor agonist, (+)-4-propyl-9-hydroxynaphthoxazine ((+)-PHNO), and discusses whether, using modern drug delivery technology, it might fill gaps in our therapeutic armory for the on–off dyskinesia syndrome of Parkinson's disease.

BASIC PHARMACOLOGY OF (+)-PHNO

The (+) enantiomer of (+)-PHNO is structurally different from other dopamine agonists, which are morphine or ergot derivatives.

A wide range of in vitro and in vivo techniques has been used to study (+)-PHNO and to define its spectrum of pharmacological activity (13). The enantiomers of PHNO has been compared with standard dopamine agonists to determine their ability to inhibit the in vitro bindings of ^{3}H-apomorphine to homogenates of rat striatal membranes (see reference 13). In this test, (+)-PHNO was more potent than bromocriptine but less potent than apomorphine, lisuride, or pergolide. (−)-PHNO is essentially devoid of activity, thus defining (+)-PHNO as the enantiomer possessing dopamine agonist activity. Because (+)-PHNO fails to stimulate adenylate cyclase activity in carp retina (13) it is further classified as a D-2 dopamine agonist (according to the criteria of Kebabian and Calne (14)). The distinction between D-1 and D-2 activity is based on the results of in vitro activity and its significance in therapeutics remains uncertain; however, present evidence indicates that D-2 agonist activity is necessary for a drug to be effective in Parkinson's disease.

Dopamine agonist activity has also been assessed in vivo by studying the ability of (+)-PHNO to produce the following effects: hypothermia in mice, postural asymmetrics in unilaterally caudectomized mice, stereotypies in rats, rotation in 6-hydroxydopamine-lesioned rats and emesis in beagles (13, 15, 16). In each of these models (+)-PHNO was compared with apomorphine and other dopamine agonists.

In comparisons of the relative doses of dopamine agonists required to produce stereotyped behavior in rats (gnawing, licking, sniffing), (+)-PHNO is the most potent (13). The ability of (+)-PHNO to evoke stereotypy in rats can be clocked by pretreatment with haloperidol but not with an alpha-methylparatyrosine (a tyrosine hydroxylase inhibitor) or reserpine (an amine-depleting agent). In rats with unilateral 6-hydroxydopamine lesions, (+)-PHNO produces turning away from the side of the lesion due to stimulation of the supersensitive dopamine receptors in the striatum deprived of its nigral input (13, 16). These results imply that (+)-PHNO is a directly acting postsynaptic dopamine agonist. It has been shown to be effective when given orally, intravenously, or by intraperitoneal injection (13, 16).

In all the in vivo models (+)-PHNO was more potent than any of the standard dopamine agonists with which it was compared (13, 16). However, this differs from the relative potencies of these drugs when tested in vitro (13, 16). The discrepancy may reflect a weakness in the in vitro model, although for other drugs it seems to be a reliable predictor of the in vivo activity (15). Alternatively, it is possible that (+)-PHNO is converted in the living animals to an active metabolite with even greater potency.

The affinity of (+)-PHNO for other receptors has been tested by measuring its ability to inhibit the binding of specific ligands to appropriate brain tissue homogenates (13, 16). That is, (+)-PHNO exhibits low IC_{50} levels for ^3H-apomorphine and ^3H-spiperone, reflecting the high affinity of (+)-PHNO for dopamine and "neuroleptic" receptors, as expected of a dopamine agonist. (+)-PHNO also has some affinity for serotonin -1 receptors (5HT-1) or alpha-2 receptors but not for other receptors to any significant extent.

The ratio of receptor affinities gives a measure of in vitro selectivity, which in the case of (+)-PHNO is 11.4 for 5HT-1/dopamine and 3.5 for an alpha-2/dopamine (16). A measure of in vivo selectivity can also be derived by comparing biological effects thought to be specific for a certain receptor class (for example, mydriasis in rats for alpha-2 receptors, stereotypy in rats for dopamine receptors).

In comparing the selectivities of (+)-PHNO for 5HT and alpha-2 receptors by in vitro and in vivo methods, with other dopamine agonists, apomorphine is the most selective dopamine agonist known and has very little action on 5HT or alpha-2 receptors. Lisuride has very little alpha-2 action but is known to act as a 5HT agonist.

Comparison between the receptor selectivity ratios of (+)-PHNO and pergolide is also of interest. Pergolide seems to be more selective than (+)-PHNO when tested in vitro but less selective in vivo. A similar difference between the potency of (+)-PHNO in vitro and in vivo was noted earlier. This discrepancy may be due to an incompatibility between the experimental models or the possibility that a more potent metabolite is at work.

NEW DRUG DELIVERY TECHNOLOGIES FOR THE CENTRAL NERVOUS SYSTEM

One of the biotechnology fields that is beginning to have a significant impact on neuropharmacology is that of new drug delivery systems. In recent years, drug delivery technology has made some exciting strides beyond the traditional forms of drugs in tablets and capsules or parenteral injection formulations. New drug delivery systems are being developed to achieve rate-controlled, targeted delivery to the central nervous system to ensure not only that a therapeutic agent gets into the central nervous system, but that it does so at the right dose and at the desired rate (17–20).

(+)-PHNO IN PARKINSON'S DISEASE

Previous investigations have shown that (+)-PHNO is effective in acutely reversing the features of Parkinson's disease (21, 22). It does this both in recently diagnosed patients with a stable response to levodopa, and in patients with more long-standing disease who exhibit fluctuations.

However, these clinical trials suggest that a single oral dose of (+)-PHNO will not act for much longer than 2 hours. This relatively short duration of action of (+)-PHNO in its present form (a conventional oral dosage formulation) might limit its usefulness. However, there is increasing evidence that continuous drug delivery is of benefit to patients with Parkinson's disease. It has been shown that a continuous intravenous levodopa infusion can abolish motor fluctuations, and there have been various attempts to adapt this concept for practical use.

Oral slow-release drug formulations are now becoming increasingly sophisticated (23). It is possible that the development of (+)-PHNO along similar lines may improve the therapeutic response to this drug by achieving constant plasma levels.

To test the effectiveness of this concept, we have emulated such a delivery method by conducting a trial of (+)-PHNO administered by continuous nasogastric infusion. Six patients with Parkinson's disease (mean duration of illness, 11.8 years) were studied who all showed on–off fluctuations in response to their normal levodopa therapy. The patients received no antiparkinsonian drugs overnight, and at the beginning of each infusion they were always off. Their response was then measured as the amount of time spent on during the infusion, which continued for 4 to 8 hours without any concurrent levodopa. Our results show a relationship between time spent on and total dose of (+)-PHNO, thus confirming the results of Grandas-Perez et al. (22).

But in addition, we have shown that patients spent a higher proportion of the infusion time on with higher infusion rates (Figure 1). Four patients received prolonged nasogastric infusions that continued all day and overnight (the longest being 79 hours). They also took Sinemet or Madopar concurrently as required. During these (+)-PHNO infusions all four patients spent a greater proportion of their waking hours on, despite receiving much smaller doses of levodopa. As an alternative to oral sustained release formulations, it may also become possible to administer (+)-PHNO to patients using transdermal delivery devices, a possibility under current investigation.

In conclusion, new advances in the treatment of the on–off dyskinesia syndrome of Parkinson's disease may provide useful clues for the understanding of the TD syndrome.

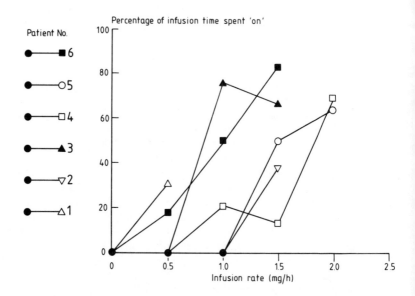

Figure 1. The response of on–off patients to increasing infusion rates of nasogastric (+)-PHNO.

REFERENCES

1. Marsden CD, Parkes JD: "On–off" effects in patients with Parkinson's disease on chronic levodopa therapy. Lancet 1:292–296, 1976

2. Melamed E: Initiation of levodopa therapy in Parkinsonian patients should be delayed until the advanced stages of the disease. Arch Neurol 43:402–405, 1986

3. Markham CH, Diamond SG: Evidence to support early levodopa therapy in Parkinson's disease. Neurology 31:125–131, 1981

4. Rinne UK: Combined bromocriptine–levodopa therapy early in Parkinson's disease. Neurology 35:1196–1198, 1985

5. Lees AJ, Stern G: Sustained bromocriptine therapy in previously untreated patients with Parkinson's disease. J Neurol Neurosurg Psychiatry 44:1020–1022, 1981

6. Quinn N, Parkes JD, Marsden CE: Control of on/off phenomenon by continuous intravenous infusion of levodopa. Neurology (Cleveland) 34:1131–1136, 1984

7. Hardie RJ, Lees AJ, Stern G: On–off fluctuations in Parkinson's disease. Brain 107:487–506, 1984

8. Nutt JG, Woodward WR, Hammerstad JP, et al: The "on–off" phenomenon in Parkinson's disease. N Engl J Med 310:483–488, 1984

9. Quinn NP, Marion M, Marsden CD: An open study of Madopar HBS, a new formulation of levodopa with benserazide, in thirteen patients with Parkinson's disease and on–off fluctuations. Eur Neurol (in press)

10. Cooper DR, Marrel C, Testa B, et al: L-Dopa methyl ester—a candidate for chronic systemic delivery of L-dopa in Parkinson's disease. Clin Neuropharmacol 7:89–98, 1984

11. Obeso JA, Luquin MR, Martinez-Lage JM: Intravenous lisuride corrects oscillations of motor performance in Parkinson's disease. Ann Neurol 19:31–35, 1986

12. Critchley P, Grandas-Perez F, Quinn N, et al: Psychosis and the lisuride pump. Lancet 2:349, 1986

13. Martin GE, Williams M, Pettibone DJ, et al: Pharmacologic profile of a novel potent direct-acting dopamine agonist (+)-4-propyl-9-hydroxynaphthoxazine ((+)-PHNO). J Pharmacol Exp Ther 230:569–576, 1984

14. Kebabian JW, Calne DB: Multiple receptors for dopamine. Nature 277:93–96, 1979

15. Martin GE, Williams M, Haubrich DR: A pharmacological comparison of 6,7-dihydroxy-2-dimethylaminotetralin (TL-99) and Nn-propyl-3-(3-hydroxyphenyl) piperidine with (3-PPP) selected dopamine agonists. J Pharmacol Exp Ther 223:298–304, 1982

16. Martin GE, Williams M, Pettibone DJ, et al: Selectivity of (+)-4-propyl-9-hydroxynaphthoxazine ((+)-PHNO)for dopamine receptors *in vitro* and *in vivo*. J Pharmacol Exp Ther 233:395–401, 1985

17. Goldman P: Rate-controlled drug delivery. N Engl J Med 307:286–290, 1982

18. Urquhart J, Gara JW, Willis KL: Rate-controlled delivery systems in drug and hormone research. Annu Rev Pharmacol Toxicol 24:199–236, 1984

19. Obeso JA, Luquin MR, Martinez-Lage JM: Lisuride infusion pump: a device for the treatment of motor fluctuation in Parkinson's disease. Lancet 1:467–470, 1986

20. Shaw JE, Chandrasekaran SK: Controlled topical delivery of drugs for systemic action. Drug Metabol Rev 8:223–233, 1978

21. Stoessl AJ, Mak E, Calne DB: (+)-4-Propyl-9-hydroxy-naphthoxazine (PHNO), a new dopaminomimetic, in treatment of parkinsonism. Lancet 2:1330–1331, 1985

22. Grandas-Perez FJ, Jenner J, Nomoto M, et al: (+)-4-propyl-9-hydroxynaphthoxazine in Parkinson's disease. Lancet 1:906, 1986

23. Stahl S: Applications of new drug delivery technologies to Parkinson's disease and dopaminergic agents. J Neur Trans M (in press)

Chapter 17

Novel Atypical Antipsychotic Compounds: Recent Developments in the Treatment of Schizophrenia

Wim M. A. Verhoeven, M.D., Ph.D.
Johans A. Den Boer, M.D.

Chapter 17

Novel Atypical Antipsychotic Compounds: Recent Developments in the Treatment of Schizophrenia

Drug treatment of schizophrenic psychoses is based on the hypothesis that a dopaminergic (DA) hyperactivity in specific limbic brain structures, particularly the nucleus accumbens, plays a key role in the pathogenesis of these disorders. The assumption of a pathogenetic role of DA systems stems from the observation of amphetamine-induced psychosis, the central DA activity enhancing effects of this drug, and the association of antipsychotic effects with the DA blocking action of most neuroleptics in current use (1). A feature of most, if not all, classical antipsychotic compounds is that they block DA receptor systems in the central nervous system (CNS) nonselectively and that they also interact with other non-DA receptor systems (2). The fact that antipsychotic compounds neither are receptor specific, nor bind selectively to DA structures in the CNS explains the frequent occurrence of unwanted side effects, most likely those related to the extrapyramidal system, for example, parkinsonian-like symptoms and tardive dyskinesia.

The discovery in the early 1970s of specific opiate binding sites in brain tissues and the isolation of endogenous substances with morphine-like actions, the so-called endorphins, has led to several hypotheses in which disturbances in these central peptide systems are assumed to be related to various psychopathological disorders, including schizophrenia. Extensive animal experiments have subsequently suggested that the nonopiate fragments of γ-endorphin (BE 1-17), the γ-type endorphins des-tyrl-γ-endorphin (DTγE; BE 2-17) and des-enkephalin-γ-endorphin (DEγE; BE 6-17), may have

245

antipsychotic properties in humans without inducing motor side effects associated with DA receptor blocking (3, 4).

In addition, novel antipsychotic compounds, the so-called atypical neuroleptics, have been developed that have more regional specificity and a more selective effect on DA receptor systems, suggesting antipsychotic properties and less propensity to induce motor side effects (5). In this chapter we discuss the interactions between DA receptor systems and γ-type endorphins and atypical neuroleptics, respectively. The results of clinical studies with both types of compounds are also discussed.

γ-TYPE ENDORPHINS

In a number of animal behavioral tests, for example, facilitation of pole-jumping avoidance behavior, induction of grasping responses, and inhibition of apomorphine-induced decrease of locomotion, it appears that γ-endorphin and the nonopiate fragments DTγE and DEγE produce effects that are in several aspects comparable to those of neuroleptic drugs such as haloperidol (3, 4). This is in contrast to the α-endorphin (BE 1-16) and its nonopiate fragment des-Tyrl-α-endorphin (DTαE; BE 2-16), which elicit behavior similar in certain aspects to those of psychostimulant drugs such as amphetamine, which can evoke symptoms resembling schizophrenia (6). These observations led to the hypothesis that the neuroleptic-like γ-type endorphins DTγE and DEγE could be regarded as endogenous substances with antipsychotic properties, and that a functional deficiency of these neuropeptides, for example, due to a disturbed balance between α, β, and γ-type endorphins, may be implicated in the pathogenesis of schizophrenia (7).

In addition to these behavioral effects of γ-type endorphins, the influences of these peptides on brain DA systems were extensively investigated, and the results used to compare, and if possible to relate, the γ-type endorphin hypothesis with the DA hypothesis of schizophrenia. It was found that DTγE decreases the α-methylparatyrosine-induced DA depletion in some brain areas that do not include the nucleus accumbens, an effect which is similar although less widespread than that of haloperidol. These results are opposite to those reported for α-endorphin (8). Further experiments, focused on the interaction between γ-type endorphins and the directly (apomorphine) or indirectly (amphetamine) acting DA mimetics, showed that while these peptides did not interfere with the behavioral effects elicited by high doses of apomorphine and amphetamine, they antagonized in a dose-dependent manner the hypoactivity induced by low doses of apomorphine injected either systemically or directly into the nucleus accumbens. These findings suggest that γ-type endorphins interfere with presynaptically located self-inhibiting DA receptor systems, particularly in the nucleus accumbens. This effect was mimicked by low doses of the classical neuroleptic haloperidol and the atypical neuroleptic sulpiride. In addition, haloperidol antagonized the effects of high doses of apomorphine, which presumably acts via an interaction with the postsynaptically located DA receptor systems; thus γ-type endorphins may interact with certain presumably presynaptically located DA receptor systems in the nucleus accumbens that are sensitive for low doses of both DA agonists and antagonists. The fact that these peptides did not interfere with postsynaptically located nucleus caudatus DA receptors may suggest that they are devoid of extrapyramidal side effects (9, 10).

Further studies were conducted to ascertain whether these peptides are involved in the regulation of γ-type-endorphin-sensitive DA receptor systems in the nucleus accumbens. Subchronic treatment with DEγE potentiated the effects of low doses of apomorphine, suggesting an increased sensitivity of the presynaptically located DA receptor systems. Chronic intra-accumbal administration of DEγE resulted in decreased locomotion, while chronic administration of γ-endorphin antiserum induced hyperlocomotion that outlasted the treatment. These results suggest that γ-type endorphins are involved in the modulation of the setpoint for feedback regulation in neurons equipped with γ-type-endorphin-sensitive DA receptor systems (11) and imply that a chronic deficiency of γ-type endorphins could eventually lead to a subsensitivity of γ-type-endorphin-sensitive DA receptor systems (11) resulting in a sustained increase of DA release and activity. Accordingly, chronic treatment with these peptides could lead to a decreased activity of the mesolimbic DA system, thus linking the γ-type endorphin and the DA hypothesis of schizophrenia (12).

The hypothesis that schizophrenia is associated with a functional deficiency of the neuroleptic-like γ-type endorphins has stimulated considerable clinical research. In several trials, in which patients were treated with either DTγE or DEγE (43 and 36 subjects, respectively) we observed both a clinically relevant reduction of psychotic symptoms (50 percent) and a lack of side effects of an extrapyramidal nature. Usually, the peptides were administered intramuscularly [1 mg/day (DTγE) or 3 mg/day (DEγE)] for 8 to 10 days; the design of all studies, except one, was double blind, either placebo controlled or cross-over (13–17). When patients responded to treatment, the effect started after 3 to 7 days of active therapy, and all symptoms including both positive and negative decreased (18–21).

Other researchers have also investigated the effects of γ-type endorphins in schizophrenia; in 10 trials, 6 open and 4 controlled, including a total of 93 patients, a favorable response to treatment was found in only 24 subjects (Table 1). The less favorable outcome as compared to our studies may be due among other possibilities to the characteristics of the patients selected. In fact, patients suffering from chronic or residual type of schizophrenia who had been treated with relatively high doses of neuroleptics appear to be less responsive to treatment with γ-type endorphins. The work of Kissling et al. (22, 23) who treated 30 acute schizophrenic inpatients (double-blind design) for 4 weeks with either DEγE or haloperidol showing that after 14 days of treatment the mean improvement in both treatment groups was approximately the same, suggests that DEγE and halo-peridol may possibly be equipotent with respect to their antipsychotic efficacy. The study of Azorin et al. (24), which included 93 schiz-ophrenic patients with an acute exacerbation, also indicates that in patients receiving 10 mg DEγE per day (intramuscularly for four weeks), a significant decrease in psychotic symptomatology was ob-served without noticeable adverse reactions. In the case of existing motor disturbances such as parkinsonism or tardive dyskinesia, γ-type endorphins do not appear to influence the severity of these symptoms (25, 26); the induction of such symptoms by γ-type en-dorphins has not been observed.

In two studies (in neuroleptic-free patients) we investigated the effects of DTγE on the central dopamine, noradrenaline, and sero-tonin systems, and on the pituitary function (14, 16). Although we failed to observe changes on either the cerebrospinal fluid levels of homovanillic acid (HVA), methoxyhydroxyphenylglycol, and 5-hy-droxyindoleacetic acid, or the daily pattern of plasma levels of growth hormone and cortisol, we found a small but significant decrease of plasma prolactin levels.

Our results, from both animal and human studies, suggest that γ-type endorphins possess antipsychotic properties, probably without affecting the nigrostriatal DA system. The latter is supported by the findings that DTγE does not influence cerebrospinal fluid HVA levels in patients and that these peptides do not appear to induce motor side effects or affect already existing movement disorders.

It should be emphasized, however, that this work is still contro-versial, and considerable research is needed before a more definitive assessment of the neuropeptide treatment strategy for schizophrenia can be made (27).

ATYPICAL NEUROLEPTICS

The results of animal experiments would indicate that atypical neuroleptics such as clozapine and the substituted benzamides have a degree of affinity for DA systems in the mesolimbic or mesocortical areas and show more receptor selectivity compared to classical neuroleptics (28).

In the search for selective DA antagonists it has been shown that several substituted benzamides can block rat central DA receptors, for example, sulpiride, remoxipride, and raclopride (29, 30). The most extensively studied of these compounds, sulpiride, inhibits apomorphine-induced climbing behavior in the rat, causes an increase in prolactin level, and increases DA turnover in the striatum and mesolimbic systems. In certain aspects sulpiride differs from classic neuroleptics: It fails to induce catalepsy, inhibit apomorphine-induced stereotyped behavior, or inhibit DA-stimulated adenylatecyclase. The latter supports the hypothesis that sulpiride, like remoxipride, selectively blocks postsynaptically located D-2 receptors. In addition, there is some evidence that in low dosage, sulpiride might also induce presynaptic receptor blockade (31). In acute as well as in chronic schizophrenic patients, the antipsychotic efficacy of sulpiride has been suggested to be comparable to that of classic neuroleptics (28).

Results from animal experiments indicate that remoxipride causes a preferential blockade of the mesolimbic DA receptors; since this compound does not block DA-stimulated adenylatecyclase activity it has been suggested it acts selectively on D-2 receptors. Furthermore, and in contrast to most classical neuroleptics, remoxipride does not block α- and β-adrenergic, serotonergic, histaminergic, or muscarinic receptors in vitro (29, 30). Thus it appears that remoxipride and the newly developed analogue raclopride may have antipsychotic properties and a reduced risk of inducing extrapyramidal symptoms (EPS) (30, 32, 33). Remoxipride increases plasma prolactin in healthy volunteers (34), and in psychotic patients a peak increase of plasma hormone occurred 1 hour after drug intake (35). Preliminary studies with raclopride suggest that this compound affects plasma prolactin similarly (36).

Plasma HVA, known to show a decrease after administration of classic neuroleptics (37), has been found to remain unchanged (38) or to decrease (37) after either remoxipride or raclopride. So far, eight open clinical studies including 103 patients have been reported

Table 1. Clinical studies with des-tyrosine-γ-endorphin (DTγE) in schizophrenia.

Author	Design	n	Nonresponders	Responders[a]	Remarks[b]
Bourgeois et al. (40)	Open	14	12	2	Chronic patients; response in patients with short recent episode
Casey et al. (25)	Open	9	9	0	Chronic patients
Emrich et al. (41, 42)	Double-blind cross-over	13	7	6	More effect in acute than in chronic patients
Fink et al. (43)	Double-blind	7	3	4	Transient improvement in 3 patients; long-lasting effect in 1 patient
Korsgaard et al. (26)	Open	4	4	0	Chronic patients with tardive dyskinesia
Manchanda and Hirsch (44)	Open	11	9	2	Response in patients with psychotic episode in last 6 months
Meltzer et al. (45, 46)	Open	15	6	9	Greater effect in younger patients
Tamminga et al (47)	Double-blind	5	5	0	Chronic patients

Table 1. (continued)

Author	Design	n	Nonresponders	Responders[a]	Remarks[b]
Volavka et al. (48)	Double-blind cross-over	9	8	1	Severe symptoms; high doses of neuroleptics used
Mizuki et al. (49)	Single-blind	6	6	0	Chronic patients with primarily negative symptoms and treatment history with high doses of neuroleptics
Total		93	69	24	

[a]From the group of responders, 10 patients improved slightly to moderately (20 to 50 percent response), while the other patients (14) responded moderately to markedly (>50 percent response). Response is expressed as percentage decrease of baseline symptomatology.
[b]No clear definition has been given by the different authors for the terms *acute* and *chronic*.

Table 2. Open clinical studies with remoxipride in schizophrenia.

Author	Dosage (mg/day)	Duration of treatment (weeks)	n	Responders[a]	Nonresponders	Main side effects
McCready et al. (50)	60–300	4	18	9	9	Headache, sleep disorder, and somnolence in some patients
Lindstrom et al. (51)	60–300	6	10	5	5	Drowsiness and sleep disturbance in some patients
Lindstrom et al. (52)	300–600	6	6	3	3	Mild extrapyramidal symptoms in 1 patient
Devaney et al. (53)	75–300	4	15	3[b]	12	Sleep disorder in 3 patients
Mertens and De Wilde (54)	75–600	6	10	8	2	Tiredness and drowsiness in 1 patient
Laursen and Gerlach (55)	300–1200	6	14	7	7	2 cases with skin reaction; in 4 patients slight extrapyramidal symptoms
Chouinard and Turnier (56)	50–500	6	20	10[c]	10	Some cases of akathisia, fatigue, and insomnia
Den Boer et al. (38)	150–450	6	10	6	4	Mild akathisia in 4 patients

[a]Defined as those who showed a clinically relevant improvement (response > 50 percent according to the Brief Psychiatric Rating Scale.
[b]Response calculated according to the Krawiecka Scale.
[c]Response calculated according to the Clinical Global Impression.

with remoxipride (Table 2) and only one with raclopride (39); as seen from Table 2, a clinically relevant antipsychotic effect was observed in 51 patients. In the open study with raclopride, 7 out of 10 patients improved considerably (39). Side effects of treatment with remoxipride, in only a few patients, were mild and included parkinsonism and/or akathisia.

CONCLUSION

A reduction of psychotic symptoms has been reported in a substantial number of schizophrenic patients treated with either γ-type endorphins or remoxipride. Treatment with γ-type endorphins, at the dosages used, has not produced motor side effects of extrapyramidal origin. The interpretation of the available clinical results with γ-type endorphins, however, is still a matter of debate and requires further investigation.

The pharmacological profile of remoxipride and its analogs suggests that these compounds have a reduced risk of including EPS, which is in agreement with the available clinical data revealing the occurrence of mild EPS only in a limited number of patients.

In conclusion, the development of atypical neuroleptics during the last decade offers new possibilities to treat schizophrenic disorders, but long-term studies are needed to assess their efficacy and likelihood of side effects.

REFERENCES

1. Carlton PL. Manowitz P: Dopamine and schizophrenia: an analysis of theory. Neurosci Biobehav Rev 8:137–151, 1984

2. Ungerstedt, U, Herrera-Marschitz M, Forster C: Neuroleptic drugs and their action on different neuronal pathways. J Clin Psychiatry 46:34–37, 1985

3. De Wied D, Kovacs GL, Bohus B, et al: Neuroleptic activity of the neuropeptide B-LPH 62-77 ((des-tyrl)-γ-endorphin; DTγE). Eur J Pharmacol 49:427–436, 1978

4. De Wied, D, Van Ree JM, Greven HM: Neuroleptic-like activity of peptides related to (des-tyrl)-γ-endorphin: structure activity studies. Life Sci 26:1575–1579, 1980

5. Tamminga CA: Atypical neuroleptics and novel antipsychotic drugs, in Neuroleptics: Neurochemical, Behavioral and Clinical Perspectives. Edited by Coyle JT, Enna SJ. New York, Raven Press, 1983, pp. 281–295

6. Van Ree JM, Bohus B, De Wied D: Similarity between behavioral effects of des-tyrosine-γ-endorphin and haloperidol and of α-endorphin and amphetamine, in Endogenous and Exogenous Opiate Agonists and Antagonists. Edited by Leong Way E. New York, Pergamon Press, 1980, pp. 459–462

7. De Wied D: Psychopathology as a neuropeptide dysfunction, in Characteristics and Function of Opioids. Edited by Van Ree JM, Terenius L. Amsterdam, Elsevier/North-Holland Biomedical Press, 1978, pp. 113–122

8. Versteeg DHG, De Kloet ER, De Wied D: Effects of α-endorphin, β-endorphin (des-tyrl)-γ-endorphin on α-MPT-induced catecholamine disappearance in discrete regions of the rat brain. Brain Res 179:85–93, 1979

9. Van Ree JM, Innemee H, Louwerens JW, et al: Non-opiate β-endorphin fragments and dopamine—I. The neuroleptic-like γ-endorphin fragments interfere with behavioral effects elicited by small doses of apomorphine. Neuropharmacology 21:1095–1101, 1982

10. Van Ree JM, Caffe AM, Wolterink G: Non-opiate β-endorphin fragments and dopamine—III. γ-Type endorphins and various neuroleptics counteract the hypoactivity elicited by injection of apomorphine into the nucleus accumbens. Neuropharmacology 21:1111–1117, 1982

11. Van Ree JM, Wolterink G, Fekete M, et al: Non-opiate β-endorphin fragments and dopamine—IV. γ-Type endorphins may control dopaminergic systems in the nucleus accumbens. Neuropharmacology 21:1119–1127, 1982

12. Van Ree JM, De Wied D: Neuroleptic-like profile of γ-type endorphins as related to schizophrenia. Trends in Pharmacological Sciences 3:358–361, 1982

13. Verhoeven WMA, Van Praag HM, Van Ree JM, et al: Improvement of schizophrenic patients by treatment with (des-tyrl)-γ-endorphin (DTγE). Arch Gen Psychiatry 36:294–298, 1979

14. Verhoeven WMA, Westenberg HGM, Gerritsen AW, et al: (Des-tyrosine)-γ-endorphin in schizophrenia: clinical, biochemical and hormonal aspects. Psychiatry Res 5:293–309, 1981

15. Verhoeven WMA, Van Ree JM, Heezius-an Bentum A, et al: Antipsychotic properties of (des-enkephalin)-γ-endorphin (DEγE; β-LPH 66-77) in schizophrenic patients. Arch Gen Psychiatry 39:648–654, 1982

16. Verhoeven WMA, Van Ree JM, Westenberg HGM, et al: Clinical biochemical and hormonal aspects of treatment with des-tyrl-γ-endorphin in schizophrenia. Psychiatry Res 11:329–346, 1984

17. Verhoeven WMA, Westenberg HGM, Van Ree JM: A comparative study on the antipsychotic properties of desenkephalin-γ-endorphins and ceruletide in schizophrenic patients. Acta Psychiatr Scand 37:372–382, 1986

18. Verhoeven WMA, Van Ree JM, Verhey FH, et al: The antipsychotic and neuroleptic-like action of γ-type endorphins, in Psychopharmacology: Impact on Clinical Psychiatry. Edited by Morgan DW. St. Louis, Ishiyaku Euro American, 1985, pp. 73–98

19. Verhoeven WMA, Van Ree JM, De Wied D: Neuroleptic-like peptides in schizophrenia, in Handbook on Studies in Schizophrenia. Edited by Burrows GD, Norman TR, Rubinstein G. Amsterdam, Elsevier Science Publishers, 1986, pp. 253–267

20. Van Ree JM, Verhoeven WMA, De Wied D: Antipsychotic actions of the endorphins, in Antipsychotics. Edited by Burrows GD, Norman TR, Davies B. Amsterdam, Elsevier Science Publishers, 1985, pp. 27–46

21. Van Ree JM, Verhoeven WMA, Claas FHJ, et al: Antipsychotic action of γ-type endorphins: animal and human studies. Prog Brain Res 1986, 65:221–235

22. Kissling W, Moller HJ, Bork F, et al: Multicenter double-blind comparison between des-enkephalin-γ-endorphin (DEγE, Org. 5878) and haloperidol concerning the efficacy and safety in the treatment of schizophrenia. Presented at the 14th Collegium Internationale Neuropsychopharmalogicum, Florence, 1984

23. Kissling W, Moller JH, Cootjans J, et al: Multicenter double-blind comparison between des-enkephalin-γ-endorphin (DEγE, Org. 5878) and haloperidol concerning the efficacy and safety in the treatment of schizophrenia, in Psychiatry and Its Related Disciplines: The Next 25 Years. Copenhagen, Denmark, World Psychiatric Association, 1986, p. 178

24. Azorin JM, Charbaut J, Granier F, et al: Des-enkephalin-gamma-endorphin in exacerbation of chronic schizophrenia: double-blind, placebo-controlled study. Presented at Neuropeptides and Brain Function Meeting, Utrecht, 1986

25. Casey DE, Korsgaard S, Gerlach J et al: Effects of destyrosine-γ-endorphin in tardive dyskinesia. Arch Gen Psychiatry 38:158–160, 1981

26. Korsgaard S, Casey DE, Gerlach J: High-dose destyrosine-γ-endorphin in tardive dyskinesia. Psychopharmacology 78:285–286, 1982

27. Nemeroff CB, Berger PA, Bissette G: Peptides in schizophrenia, in Psychopharmacology: The Third Generation of Progress. Edited by Meltzer H. New York, Raven Press, 1986, pp. 727–745

28. Peselow ED, Stanley M: Clinical trials of benzamide in psychiatry, in The Benzamides: Pharmacology, Neurobiology and Clinical Aspects. Edited by Stanley M, Rotrosen J. New York, Raven Press, 1982, pp. 163–194

29. Ogren SO, Hall H, Kohler O, et al: Remoxipride: a new potential antipsychotic compound with selective antidopaminergic actions in the rat brain. Eur J Pharmacol 102:459–474, 1984

30. Ogren SO, Hall H, Kohler O, et al: The selective dopamine D2 receptor antagonist raclopride discriminates between dopamine-mediated motor functions. Psychopharmacology 90:287–294, 1986

31. Worms P: Behavioral pharmacology of the benzamides as compared to standard neuroleptics, in The Benzamides: Pharmacology, Neurobiology and Clinical Aspects. Edited by Stanley M, Rotrosen J. New York, Raven Press, 1982, pp. 7–16

32. Kohler C, Hall H, Ogren SO, et al: Specific in vitro and in vivo binding of ^{3}H-raclopride: a potent substituted benzamide drug with high affinity for dopamine D2-receptors in the rat brain. Biochem Pharmacol 34:2251–2259, 1985

33. Farde L, Hall H, Ehrin E, et al: Quantitative analysis of D2 dopamine receptor binding in the living human brain by PET. Science 231:258–261, 1986

34. Nillson NI, Farde L, Grind M, et al: Pharmacokinetics and effects on plasma prolactin levels of remoxipride—a new potential neuroleptic drug. Presented at the Fourth World Congress on Biologic Psychiatry, Philadelphia, PA, 1985

35. Chouinard G, Turnier L, Kallai-Sanfacon MA; Remoxipride in schizophrenia: effects on plasma prolactin. Prog Neuropsychopharmacol Biol. Psychiatry 9:599–603, 1985

36. Wahlen A, Farde L, Wiesel FA, et al: Biochemical effects of the potential antipsychotic drug raclopride in schizophrenic patients. Presented at International Union of Pharmacology Symposium, Sydney, 1987

37. Pickar D, Labarea R, Linnoila M, et al: Neuroleptic-induced decrease in plasma homovanillic acid and antipsychotic activity in schizophrenic patients. Science 225:954–956, 1984

38. Den Boer JA, Verhoeven WMA, Westenberg HGM: Remoxipride in schizophrenia: a preliminary report. Acta Psychiatr Scand 74:409–414, 1986

39. Farde L. Wiesel FA, Oxenstierna G, et al: Raclopride: a new potential antipsychotic compound. Presented at the 15th Collegium Internationale Neuropsychopharmacologicum, Puerto Rico, 1986

40. Bourgeois M, Laforge E, Muyard J, et al: Endorphines et schizophrenies. Ann Med Psychol 138:1112–1119, 1980

41. Emrich HM, Zaudig M, Kissling W, et al: Des-tyrosyl-γ-endorphin in schizophrenia: a double-blind trial in 13 patients. Pharmacopsychiatry 13:290–298, 1980

42. Emrich HM, Zaudig M, Von Zerssen D, et al: Action of (des-tyrl)-γ-endorphin in schizophrenia. Mod Probl Pharmacopsychiatry 17:279–286, 1981

43. Fink M, Papakostas Y, Lee J, et al: Clinical trials with des-tyr-gamma-endorphin (GK-78), in Biological Psychiatry. Edited by Perris C, Struwe G, Jansson B. Amsterdam, Elsevier/North-Holland Biomedical Press, 1981, pp. 398–401

44. Manchanda R, Hirsch SR: (Des-tyrl)-γ-endorphin in the treatment of schizophrenia. Psychol Med 11:401-404, 1981

45. Meltzer HY, Busch DA, Tricou BJ, et al: Effect of (des-tyr)-gamma-endorphin in schizophrenia. Psychiatry Res 6:313–326, 1982

46. Meltzer HY, Busch DA, Lee J, et al: Effect of des-tyr-γ-endorphin in schizophrenia. Psychopharmacol Bull 18:44–47, 1982

47. Tamminga CA, Tighe PJ, Chase T, et al: Des-tyrosine-γ-endorphin administration in chronic schizophrenics. Arch Gen Psychiatry 38:167–168, 1981

48. Volavka J, Hui KS, Anderson B, et al: Short-lived effect of (des-tyr)-gamma-endorphin in schizophrenia. Psychiatry Res 10:243–252, 1983

49. Mizuki Y, Ushijima I, Yamada M, et al: A treatment trial with an analog of thyrotropin-releasing hormone (DN-1417) and des-tyrosine-γ-endorphin in schizophrenia. Int Clin Psychopharmacol 1:303–313, 1986

50. McCready RG, Morrision D, Eccleston D, et al: An open multicentre study of the treatment of florid schizophrenia with remoxipride. Acta Psychiatr Scand 72:139–143, 1985

51. Lindstrom LH, Besev G. Stening G, et al: An open study of remoxipride, a benzamide derivative, in schizophrenia. Psychopharmacology 86:241–243, 1985

52. Lindstrom LH, Besev G, Stening G, et al: The effect of remoxipride, a novel dopamine-D2 receptor blocker, in chronic schizophrenia, an open study. Presented at the Fourth World Congress Biologic Psychiatry, Philadelphia, PA, 1985

53. Devaney N, King DJ, Cooper SJ, et al: An open study of remoxipride, a new neuroleptic, in chronic schizophrenia. Presented at the Fourth World Congress on Biologic Psychiatry, Philadelphia, PA, 1985

54. Mertens C, De Wilde J: An open label, noncomparative study of remoxipride in schizophrenia. Presented at the Fourth World Congress on Biologic Psychiatry, Philadelphia, PA, 1985

55. Laursen AL, Gerlach J: Antipsychotic effect of remoxipride, a new substituted benzamide with selective antidopaminergic activity. Acta Psychiatr Scand 73:17–21, 1986

56. Chouinard G, Turnier L: An early phase II clinical trial of remoxipride in schizophrenia with measurement of plasma neuroleptic activity. Psychopharmacol Bull 22:267-271, 1986

Chapter 18

Legal Liability for Tardive Dyskinesia: Guidelines for Practice

Phyllis E. Amabile, J.D., M.D.
James L. Cavanaugh, Jr., M.D.

Chapter 18

Legal Liability for Tardive Dyskinesia: Guidelines for Practice

Although tardive dyskinesia (TD) was first described in the medical literature in the early 1960s, it has only been during the last decade that this neurological syndrome has been recognized as a serious and widespread phenomenon with enormous medical, ethical, and legal implications. The purpose of this chapter is to describe the various ways in which TD can lead to a treating physician's legal liability, to review the pertinent case law, and to provide guidelines for psychiatric practice. We shall begin with descriptions of the law of malpractice, informed consent, breach of contract, strict liability, and fraud. A brief discussion of the patient's right to refuse treatment will be followed by a consideration of special problems and common questions in treating with antipsychotic medication. We shall conclude the chapter with a discussion of the American Psychiatric Association Task Force guidelines and of potential future legal developments.

MEDICAL MALPRACTICE

Medical malpractice is a form of negligence referring to professional misconduct that consists of an unreasonable lack of skill or care in one's work. More specifically, it refers to bad or injudicious professional treatment of a patient that results in injury, suffering, or death, due to the physician's ignorance, carelessness, lack of proper skill, or disregard of established principles (1). In order for a suing injured party (plaintiff) to have a legal "cause of action" against a physician for medical malpractice, the party must prove several elements. The physician must have had a duty to the patient because of having undertaken an obligation to treat him or her, and the physician must have negligently breached the duty through some error or omission in diagnosis or treatment. The patient must have sustained some harm (physical or emotional) that is very closely related to the physician's negligence ("proximate causation") (2, 3).

In the last several years, there has been a burgeoning of suits by patients who have developed TD, based on claims of negligence. Several have resulted in large damage awards or out-of-court settlements against physicians, hospitals, and clinics. Perhaps the best known of these cases is *Clites v. Iowa*,[1] in which almost $800,000.00 was awarded to a mentally retarded young adult who had been in a state residential treatment facility since the age of 11. When the patient was 18, he was first treated with neuroleptic medications for "aggressive and sexual behavior." Several different treating physicians prescribed the medications continuously for 5 years, despite the eventual development of a fairly severe form of TD. In fact, it was the patient's parents who, upon hearing a news report about TD, realized that their son was suffering from the syndrome and demanded that the medication be stopped. The court, after hearing expert testimony on the appropriate standards of care in using antipsychotic medications, found that the defendants had been negligent in several ways. There was insufficient evidence of any severe aggression or self-abuse that would have justified prescribing the drugs in Clites's case. The staff ignored the risks of uninterrupted use of major tranquilizers and failed to monitor the patient closely. Indeed, Clites's records indicated that he had not had a physical examination or been regularly visited by a physician for 3 consecutive years. Failure of the hospital staff to react to the developing signs of TD, and the failure of the patient's attending physician, who was unfamiliar with TD, to obtain consultation with a specialist, also constituted malpractice. The court viewed the use of polypharmacy and the use of medication primarily for the convenience of the staff as substandard medical care. Finally, the failure of the hospital to inform Clites's parents of the dangers of prolonged use of neuroleptics and obtain their informed consent was negligent (4, 5).

In *Faigenbaum v. Oakland Medical Center*,[2] a 55-year-old woman who had been variously diagnosed as depressive and schizophrenic was treated with antipsychotic medication for 12 years. When TD developed, a neurologist diagnosed Huntington's chorea and recommended further antipsychotic treatment. Although other physicians made the correct diagnosis, the treating psychiatrist relied on the neurologist's diagnosis and continued neuroleptic medication. The plaintiff successfully sued several defendants, including the treating psychiatrist, and received total damages nearing $1.5 million. The court found the defendants to have been negligent in failing to accurately diagnose TD. Specifically, the judge stated that physicians had a duty to seek out the patient's prior medical records, to take a drug history, and to be aware of the contents of package inserts warning of TD. The failure to correctly diagnose led to further malpractice in that neuroleptics continued to be administered in a negligent fashion and the TD went unattended. All of these factors were judged to be below the standard of medical care.

Similarly, in *Lundgren v. Eustermann*,[3] the defendant physician was held liable for the negligent failure to carefully monitor and record the side effects of Thorazine (TD). Of interest is the fact that the defendant in this case was a family physician who continued treating the patient with Thorazine after she was discharged from the inpatient care of a psychiatrist who had begun the medication prior to her discharge from the hospital.

One final TD case is of interest because of its factual context. In *Hedin v. United States*,[4] a 36-year-old veteran had been taking Mellaril, and later Thorazine, for 4 years before TD was diagnosed. The syndrome led to the breakup of his marriage and the loss of his job. As an outpatient at a Veterans Administration Hospital, the plaintiff had not seen a physician for 17 months while his neuroleptic prescriptions were filled by the hospital through the mail. The court found the hospital physicians to have been negligent in prescribing without monitoring the patient. Over $2 million was awarded in damages.

In each of the four cases discussed above, the defendant physicians were found negligent in having fallen below the applicable standard of medical care, to which medical experts testified. How does a court determine standards of care? As a general rule, the courts hold physicians to the reasonable care and skill that would be possessed and exercised by an ordinary member of the profession of good standing under similar circumstances. The standard of competence for a psychiatrist who is a "specialist" or "expert" in some area of the field would be higher than that of the "ordinary psychiatrist."

In the course of litigation against a physician for medical malpractice, the plaintiff must offer expert testimony to establish the standard of care and the doctor's departure from that standard. In general, the witness must possess both the necessary schooling and training in the subject matter involved, as well as practical or occupational experience with the subject. Ordinarily, the expert testimony is considered by the courts to be best supplied if the expert witness is also a physician, especially one in the same area of practice, but this is not essential.

In the *Lundgren*[5] case, a licensed consulting Ph.D. psychologist with extensive training and experience in psychology and pharmacology was found to be incompetent to give an expert opinion on the standard of medical care required of the defendant family physician. This was not because the witness was a psychologist, but rather because he had never prescribed the drug in question and did not know how physicians customarily used Thorazine in treatment. Theoretical knowledge was considered insufficient.

In a few reported cases, courts have *judicially* created a standard of care contrary to the standard of the medical profession. For example, in *Helling v. Carey*,[6] the Washington State Supreme Court found defendant ophthalmologists negligent because of their failure to administer a glaucoma test to a patient under age 40 who was later partially blinded from open-angle glaucoma. This holding was despite uncontradicted expert testimony that the universal practice in the profession was not to routinely test patients younger than 40 for glaucoma.[7]

Such cases can pose a distressing dilemma for the medical profession. A physician can be held liable for negligent malpractice under a court-created standard of care despite the fact that at the time of the event giving rise to the lawsuit, he or she was conscientiously abiding by the standards of the profession. Philosophical and ethical questions also are raised when nonmedical professionals (for example, the courts) create medical standards of care. To our knowledge, there have not been to date any judicially created standards of care relating to TD.

INFORMED CONSENT

The doctrine of informed consent has developed over the last 25 years in the United States, creating a physician duty of "reasonable disclosure" in order to protect a patient's right to self-determination (3). The first U.S. case to proclaim the physician's duty to obtain informed consent was *Salgo v. Leland Stanford Jr. University*, wherein a California court declared, "A physician . . . subjects himself to liability if he withholds any facts which are necessary to form the basis of an intelligent consent by the patient" (6).[8] In part, the duty to obtain an informed consent is considered a corollary of the patient's right to refuse medication in nonemergency situations, now recognized in most states (7).

The failure of a physician to obtain an adequate informed consent prior to rendering treatment may constitute a form of negligence if harm occurs as a result of the treatment. The failure must have "caused" the harm, in that adequate disclosure of information would have led to the patient's decision to forego the treatment (3, 8).

Three main elements compose an informed consent: adequate information, voluntariness, and competency. The information a physician must disclose, known as the "elements of disclosure," consists of an explanation of the nature and purpose of the proposed treatment, the potential risks, the anticipated benefits, and the alternatives to the proposed treatment with their attendant risks and benefits. As a general rule, it is wise to inform the patient of the most common and of the most serious risks (for example, TD when treating with neuroleptics). Voluntariness implies an absence of any coercion (for example, from physicians, family, institution) that would undermine a patient's autonomy. Competency requires that the patient possess adequate mental ability to participate meaningfully in the decision making (8, 9).

How much information must a physician disclose about the proposed treatment in order for it to be considered "adequate?" The majority of courts adhere to a professional standard of disclosure, considering what disclosure is customary and usual among other reasonable, careful, and skillful members of the profession under similar circumstances. A substantial minority of courts, however, now adhere to a patient-centered standard as first articulated in the landmark *Canterbury v. Spence*[9] case in 1972. This standard questions whether the physician's disclosure of information was reasonable given what he or she knew or should have known to be the patient's informational needs. The test to ascertain whether a particular peril must be divulged is its materiality for a reasonable patient's decision.[10] The patient-centered standard was applied in the 1986 *Barclay v. Campbell*[11] case in which a patient who developed TD sued his physician for negligent failure to have disclosed that risk to him. The Texas Supreme Court reaffirmed a physician's duty to inform a patient on neuroleptics of the material risk of TD and articulated that the physician must disclose a risk which could influence a reasonable person, even if he or she believes that particular patient is not capable of making a reasonable decision. "Barclay's mental illness does not foreclose his right to be informed of the risk."[12]

When attempting to obtain an informed consent, a physician should always question and document whether there is any reason to doubt a patient's competency. Various criteria have been suggested, such as, Does the patient evidence a choice? Is the choice based on "rational" reasons? Does the patient have the ability to understand? Does the patient have actual understanding? Is the patient's choice "reasonable" (10)? When a patient appears unable to make or communicate a responsible decision, the physician should either seek substituted consent or initiate guardianship proceedings through the courts, as provided by the laws of the particular state (8). A person can technically be declared legally "incompetent" only by a court of law.

Certain exceptions to the doctrine of informed consent exist. First, if the patient is incompetent, consent must be obtained from a substitute decision maker authorized by law, as described above. Second, in an emergency situation where immediate action must be taken to prevent death or serious harm, the law considers the consent to be "implied." States vary considerably as to how narrowly they define "emergency," but as a general rule patients who are violent or threatening harm to themselves or others could be given antipsychotic medication without prior informed consent. (Note that the emergency exception applies even if the patient is incompetent.) Third, patients who understand that they have the right to be informed and to make a treatment decision can intentionally waive the right. Finally, "therapeutic privilege" allows a physician to withhold information that he or she believes would directly damage the patient or impede his or her rational decision making. The courts have upheld the privilege on rare occasions; it would behoove the treating psychiatrist to avoid invoking this privilege, especially where the nondisclosure of significant risk like TD would be involved (8, 9).

Perhaps because TD is such an unpredictable, potentially debilitating syndrome that has led to multiple lawsuits nationwide, "informed consent" for antipsychotic treatment is very complex. A number of special concerns deserve consideration here, such as physician resistance to discussing TD, patient understanding and recall, and ethical dilemmas.

Despite widespread publicity about TD in recent years, psychiatrists may still often be reluctant to discuss this risk with patients. One commentator has suggested some plausible explanations for this. It is psychologically painful for a clinician to recognize that medication he or she has prescribed may cause severe and irreversible harm. However, it is sometimes feared that information about the syndrome will destroy a fragile working alliance or invite lawsuits, especially with patients who are hostile, paranoid, or ambivalent (11).

A question is often raised as to how soon after the initiation of antipsychotic treatment consent should be obtained. Ideally, consent would be obtained prior, especially since in rare cases TD has developed after just a few weeks of treatment. The condition of acutely psychotic patients may interfere with their ability to give a truly informed consent. Many commentators believe that this justified delaying the consent procedures until the psychosis has remitted enough to allow reasonable participation. This could take anywhere from a few weeks to 6 months, but it is believed to be a sensible approach since the risk of developing TD after just a few months of treatment is low (6, 10, 12). Of course, if a patient does not regain the ability to give informed consent within a few months, steps to obtain substituted consent or guardianship should be taken. Logically, the longer a clinician treats a patient with neuroleptics, absent his or a proxy's informed consent, the greater the risk of malpractice liability.

Several studies have been done that call into question patients' ability to understand and recall information given to them by their clinicians (13–15). Jaffe (13) interviewed groups of medical and psychiatric outpatients and found both to be knowledgeable about the short-term side effects of their various medications, usually because of personal experience with them. But the knowledge of both groups was inadequate regarding potential long-term side effects. Ganguli and Raghu (14) gave detailed information about TD to schizophrenic patients on neuroleptic medications, and further instructed those with defective recall 2 weeks later. Ultimately, all patients without TD had some recall of the information, but the majority of those who had TD could not remember any discussion taking place. The authors posit some possible explanations for this surprising finding. Munetz and Roth (15) discovered that patients receiving an informal (oral) presentation about TD retained significantly more information over 2 months than patients who received a formal (written) presentation. However, neither group learned the information that the authors considered to be most relevant to decision making about the neuroleptics.

These studies raise an interesting question about whether informed consent doctrine assumes understanding and recall that is beyond many patients' capabilities. Indeed, one commentator has questioned whether informed consent guidelines have developed more to protect physicians from litigation than to protect patients from the dangers of treatment (12). Other ethical problems exist as well: For example, can a patient whose psychosis has been alleviated by medication properly consent to continuing the drug, when it is likely that discontinuing the treatment may result in refusal to consent (12)? While there is no clear, simple answer to any of these dilemmas, a treating psychiatrist's sensitivity to their existence is important.

OTHER POTENTIAL FOUNDATIONS FOR LIABILITY: BREACH OF CONTRACT, FRAUD, AND STRICT LIABILITY

The nature of the therapeutic relationship between physician and patient is a contractual one. Certain terms are "implied" by law into the contract, such as that the doctor possesses and will exercise a reasonable degree of skill and care in his or her treatment. In addition, the physician and patient may have other "express" terms in their contract (for example, frequency of sessions, fees). Were a physician to make an express promise or warranty to a patient and fail to perform the promise, he or she could be liable for breach of contract even if no negligence were involved. For example, in *Guilmet v. Campbell*,[13] surgeons who promised that an operation for relief of peptic ulcer would pose "no danger" and would "take care of all [the patient's] troubles" were liable for breach of contract when severe complications arose postoperatively. Likewise, *Johnson v. Rodis*[14] involved a physician's promise that electroconvulsive therapy was "perfectly safe," a warranty that failed when his patient suffered a fractured arm. Were a physician to state that antipsychotic medications would cure schizophrenia, or that they were without serious side effects, liability for breach of contract could ensue.

A physician who intentionally made false representations to a patient or who concealed some information that should have been disclosed could be guilty of fraud. For example, in *Simcuski v. Saeli*,[15] a physician who had negligently severed a nerve during the surgical excision of a node concealed that fact from his patient and promised that physiotherapy would produce a cure. Similarly, were a psychiatrist to misrepresent the safety or effectiveness of a neuroleptic medication, or to conceal the true nature of developing signs of TD in a patient, he or she could conceivably be liable for fraud.

During the last 20 years, a new body of "strict liability" law has developed in the courts. Strict liability makes the seller of a product bear the costs of an accident if the product is defective or unreasonably dangerous, beyond what would be contemplated by the consumer. If the product "proximately causes" an injury, the seller is liable even if his or her conduct was in no way negligent. Even if the seller exercised all possible care to avoid selling a product that is defective or unreasonably dangerous, he or she must bear the economic loss of the injury (16).

Strict liability law is a mechanism for spreading the costs of injuries such that persons who have been injured by defective products can obtain compensation without having to provide the defendant's "fault."

Various justifications for strict liability law have been suggested: It is often difficult to prove fault; the defendant is in a better position financially to bear the cost of the accidents (often by spreading the costs among all its consumers); the law is an incentive to sellers to market safer products (6, 17).

As a general rule, strict liability has only been applied against defendant manufacturers of various products (including, in some cases, makers of antipsychotic medications that have caused TD; see, for example, *Sandoz, Inc. v. Employer's Liability Assurance Corporation*[16]). Although proposals have been made to apply strict liability principles to medical and psychiatric services rendered by physicians, the courts have been reluctant to do so. Some commentators have noted, however, a certain trend in that direction through cases wherein the established medical standard of care is rejected by the court and replaced with its own judicially created medical standard of practice (6). The *Helling*[17] and *Gates*[18] cases cited previously are good examples of this trend, which only a few courts have followed. To our knowledge, no cases have been adjudicated wherein established psychiatric standards of care regarding TD have been rejected by a court in favor of its own standard.

THE RIGHT TO REFUSE TREATMENT

Many lawsuits have been brought during the last decade on behalf of involuntarily hospitalized patients who wish to refuse treatment with antipsychotic medications. A fear of side effects from the drugs, particularly tardive dyskinesia, is often cited as the main reason for treatment refusal.[19] In many jurisdictions, a competent patient, even one who has been involuntarily admitted to a psychiatric facility, has a right to refuse medications unless a "compelling state interest" overrides it. Interestingly, some statutes that specify this right to refuse treatment refer to the medications as "chemical restraints" or "pharmacological restraints." Such terms may be a reflection of the legislators' awareness of some past abuses of neuroleptic use in institutional settings. Absent a "compelling state interest" (usually an emergency), there is a right to refuse medication based on the constitutional rights to privacy (14th Amendment) and to "produce ideas" (seen by some as a derivative of the 1st Amendment).

Courts vary considerably as to what they consider a sufficient "emergency" to override a patient's right to refuse drugs. For example, some courts define an emergency as one in which patients pose a risk of imminent physical harm to themselves or another. Others have determined that a need for medication to prevent immediate further substantial deterioration of mental illness constitutes an emergency. In general, as long as a physician uses accepted professional judgment and follows established procedures, he or she may make the determination of an emergency without a court hearing.[20]

Some courts have not recognized a right of involuntarily hospitalized patients, even competent ones, to refuse drug treatment in nonemergency situations. As long as the medication is not used punitively, used for the convenience of the staff, or objected to on religious grounds, the patient may be required to take medication if the treating physician deems it appropriate.[21]

Incompetency has been discussed previously in relation to informed consent doctrine, but should be mentioned again here. Those jurisdictions that recognize a right to refuse medication commonly require a court hearing to determine whether treatment should be rendered to a patient who lacks the mental capacity to consent to it.[22] While such hearings are intended to afford consideration to the person's constitutional rights, they can unfortunately be costly and time consuming. For an excellent overview of the right to refuse treatment cases, see Taub (7).

CONSENT FORMS AND TD

Despite the fact that several states have enacted statutes requiring written informed consent for antipsychotic medication (7), it appears that the majority of commentators do not favor the routine use of written consent forms for neuroleptics. In the majority of jurisdictions, signed consent forms are not legally required and are not regularly used by physicians. If they are improperly or carelessly used, they can actually impede a physician's informing his or her patient and can strengthen a patient's claim that his or her consent was not an informed one (18, 19).

The actual composition of written consent forms is frequently flawed such that they do not discuss the particular treatment and its possible complications, they are too lengthy to be read completely, or they are to rife with technical medical or legal jargon to be comprehended. The goal of some consent forms appears to be protection of the physician; some even attempt to release physicians from all liability, even for negligence. It is not difficult to imagine the impression that a consent form composed in these ways would have upon a jury. Furthermore, the forms improperly used when the physician delegates the signing to a nonphysician staff member, foregoing his or her own conversation with the patient about risks, benefits, and alternatives (18).

The limited amount of clinical research that has been done to investigate the usefulness of consent forms supports these views. For example, one study provided information about medication and TD to two groups of schizophrenic patients who showed evidence of the disorder. The "formal group" was presented a written consent form, composed as clearly and accurately as possible, which was then reviewed by the patient and a therapist. The "informal group" only participated in discussions with the therapist, but covered the same material. Patients in the informal group appeared to learn more, and therapists reported feeling more comfortable, than in the formal group. The authors concluded that the best way to obtain meaningful informed consent is by repeated informal discussion in the context of a trusting therapeutic relationship (20).

Certain court decisions substantiate the criticisms some commentators have made about the possibilities of inappropriate content and misuse of consent forms. *Cathmer v. Hunter*[23] involved a battery lawsuit against a physician who performed a surgical hip prosthesis rather than the total hip replacement which he had described to his patient in an earlier consultation. Although the patient signed a consent form agreeing to the prosthesis, the physician never explained the form's contents to him. The court decided that this evidence should be considered by the jury in a determination of whether the patient had consented to hip prosthesis, notwithstanding the existence of the signed consent form. The plaintiff in *Siegel v. Mount Sinai Hospital of Cleveland*[24] was informed of the type of procedure proposed (general anesthesia for orthopedic surgery) but claimed to have been inadequately informed of the material risks. The court determined that a consent document signed by the patient was not conclusive evidence that he had been adequately informed of the special dangers of administering anesthesia to an asthmatic. Again, the question of whether he had truly consented was left to the jury. *Tunk v. Regents of the University of California*[25] involved a situation wherein a charitable hospital required patients to sign a consent form releasing the hospital from all negligent and wrongful acts as a condition for admission. The court declared the releases to be invalid as contrary to public policy and permitted the plaintiff's suit for negligence.

The American Psychiatric Association Task Force on Tardive Dyskinesia (21) does not favor the routine signing and witnessing of written consent for neuroleptic therapy. To routinely require written consent for such accepted, nonexperimental medicinal therapy could set a new standard-of-care precedent. Furthermore, unlike the brief, acute risks of many procedures for which limited consent can meaningfully be given, neuroleptic treatment of chronic mental disorders is often modified over long periods of time. Anything other than an undesirable "blanket" written consent would therefore be unfeasible (21).

Some commentators have indicated that written consent forms should always be used with patients who in the past have had reversible dyskinesia or who currently have signs of the disorder and require further neuroleptic therapy. They suggest that the difficulty of overgeneralization can be avoided by describing in the written consent the observed TD symptoms, their presumed relationship to the drug, the possibility of the drug's "masking" symptoms, the fact of no known effective treatment for TD, and the current need for continuing therapy (12, 22).

COMMON QUESTIONS AND GENERAL GUIDELINES FOR PRACTICE

It is important to recognize that some of the earliest TD litigation, and those cases which resulted in some of the largest damage awards, involved grossly neglectful behavior on the part of the treating physicians (for example, *Hedin v. United States*[26]). Evidence of extremely careless psychiatric practice may not only tend to lead to larger damage awards against a particular physician, but it may encourage further TD litigation as well. Therefore, it is essential that practices which could foster the development of or failure to recognize TD be avoided. Refilling prescribed antipsychotic medication automatically through the mail or by telephone for months in succession without personally examining the patient (as in the *Hedin* case) is a poor and dangerous practice. A special problem can exist when a number of physicians treat the same patient for a period of time in succession, as is commonly the case at community mental health centers or in clinics staffed by residents in training. The needs for ongoing informed consent and frequent monitoring for TD or dosage adjustments are easily overlooked.

There is some evidence that the use of antipsychotic medication in children or with the mentally retarded can also pose special problems. Many of these patients, particularly those in institutions and treated with high doses of medication for extended periods of time, have developed the disorder. At times the drugs have been used more for their "tranquilizing" action than for a specific antipsychotic effect in children or mentally retarded individuals who show behavior problems, hyperkinesis, or severe anxiety. This is despite the fact that there are few empirical data to support such clinical use of neuroleptics in nonpsychotic patients (23, 24).

Given the specific risks of TD and the dangers of malpractice litigation that could ensue, some clinicians have considered whether it is preferable to avoid the use of neuroleptic medication altogether. Studies have well documented the greater efficacy of these drugs over psychotherapy, electroconvulsive therapy, and milieu therapy in treating acute psychotic episodes and in preventing relapses (25). The failure to prescribe the medication for illnesses wherein its efficacy has been proved right might therefore be considered malpractice in itself, and raises ethical concerns as well (7, 26).

Once a psychiatrist has determined that antipsychotic medication is indicated, fully informing the patient and obtaining informed consent is necessary. If a practitioner chooses to use written consent forms, he or she must realize that they do not offer full protection from a claim of lack of informed consent. The form should specify the particular treatment with its most serious and most frequent risks, should avoid technical or overly elaborate medical and legal jargon, and should never serve as a substitute for discussion with the patient (18, 27). The primary treating physician should obtain the consent, and where feasible, the patient's family should be present as well (28). When consent forms are not used, it is crucial that the patient's records indicate highlights of the discussion that took place in obtaining informed consent. If a physician has developed a routine method of explaining the treatment, the note can indicate that the discussion was a typical one, specifying any unusual content (18). Regardless of whether consent forms are used or not, patient progress notes must indicate that the discussion of risks, benefits, and alternatives continues over time.

The concept of intermittent neuroleptic "drug holidays" has been a controversial one. At one time the practice was widely advocated, and at least one court has cited the failure to observe drug holidays as one of the bases of malpractice in a TD case (*Clites v. Iowa*[27]). However, neither clinical nor experimental data support the notion that intermittent drug therapy decreases the incidence of persistent tardive dyskinesia (10, 29, 30). It has been suggested that intermittent drug treatment may predispose patients to more severe and irreversible TD (31), but the evidence is considered inconclusive (30). Some investigators claim that drug holidays may be associated with higher rates of psychotic relapse and behavioral deterioration (32, 33). Repeated interruptions of a neuroleptic medication in a patient who needs continuous treatment as a means of preventing tardive dyskinesia is not recommended.

Other, more justifiable reasons for reducing or even periodically discontinuing a patient's medication do exist. There is some evidence that lower doses of maintenance antipsychotic drugs are associated with a lower incidence of TD (10). Reduction and discontinuation may clarify whether the patient is still in need of the medication. It may also precipitate the first observable signs of TD, previously "masked" by the drug itself. This information would be of enormous significance to the patient and physician, if only to render ongoing consent to the treatment truly "informed." It is therefore recommended that a gradual reduction of maintenance antipsychotic medication be attempted periodically for these reasons, after the patient's consent to the reduction has been obtained (30, 34).

The need for clinicians to detect cases of TD as early as possible raises the question of what method is preferred for monitoring and documenting signs of the disorder. A structured movement examination such as the Abnormal Involuntary Movement Scale (AIMS), performed at regular intervals at least every 6 months, can help one see abnormal movements previously undetected or misinterpreted. This widely used instrument is easily learned, quickly performed, and reliably scored (35). In one study, the AIMS exam took clinicians between 5 and 10 minutes to perform, some of which was spent initiating discussion with patients about TD. The exam appeared to provide a certain structure that helped the clinicians to overcome their resistances to both discussing and diagnosing TD in their patients (36).

The emergence of the first signs of TD in a patient who suffers from a severe and chronic psychotic disorder can pose a difficult ethical dilemma. (The safety of continued, long-term administration of neuroleptics to dyskinetic patients has not been determined). It is possible that the TD could worsen or that potentially reversible TD could become irreversible. Nevertheless, to discontinue needed antipsychotic medication may pose an even greater hazard to the patient. The various risks and benefits of continued treatment must be carefully evaluated with the patient's participation, and the movement disorder should be reassessed every 3 to 4 months. In this way, changes in the risk/benefit ratio can be assessed and ongoing informed consent and documentation can be more realistically achieved. In difficult cases, consultation with a neurologist or neuropsychiatrist may be advisable (12). Ideally, a gradual reduction in the dosage of medication to the point of discontinuation or "lowest effective dose" should be undertaken as soon as signs of TD appear, if this has not already been done.

The American Psychiatric Association's Task Force on Tardive Dyskinesia published a report in 1979 that suggests several excellent guidelines for the avoidance and management of TD. In summary, the Task Force's recommendations are as follows:[28]

1. The indications for prolonged antipsychotic therapy must be carefully considered, and there must be objective evidence of benefit. Long-term use is indicated in schizophrenia, paranoia, childhood psychoses, and certain neuropsychiatric disorders (such as Gilles de LaTourette's syndrome and Huntington's disease). Short-term administration (less than 6 months) is justifiable in many cases of acute psychotic episode, severe mania, depression with psychotic features, and in states of acute agitation that can occur in acute or chronic brain syndromes (such as dementia or mental retardation). In rare instances, the use of neuroleptics in patients with other conditions who have not responded to alternative treatments may be justified.
2. Alternative therapies for neuroses, mood disorders, and character disorders should be sought.
3. A clinician should use lower doses with the elderly and with children, strive for minimum effective doses, avoid multiple drugs, and discontinue antiparkinsonian agents as soon as possible.
4. After a *first* acute psychotic episode of any type has remitted, the dose of the neuroleptic should be gradually decreased and, if possible, discontinued within several months.
5. Patients and their families should be advised of risks and benefits. A mutual decision should be arrived at when the use of neuroleptics exceeds 1 year; this should be noted in the clinical record.
6. The patient should be examined regularly for early signs of TD, and alternative neurological diagnoses should be considered.
7. Every 3 to 6 months, patients should be reevaluated, indications for and responses to medication should be documented, and attempts to reduce dosage should be considered. In the case of chronically hospitalized schizophrenic patients, once or twice each year a drug withdrawal is recommended. The dosage should be reduced by about 10 percent every 3 to 7 days until discontinuation for at least 2 weeks (if clinical status permits). Such evaluations serve to detect withdrawal dyskinesia and to evaluate the need for continued drug use. This practice may also be attempted with selected outpatients.
8. At the earliest sign of TD, the clinician should lower the dose, change to a less potent agent, or, ideally, stop treatment for as long as the patient's psychiatric status permits.
9. Benign agents should first be employed to treat TD. Neuroleptics should be reinstituted for the purpose of suppressing the disorder only as an extreme measure for disabling dyskinesia.

CONCLUSION

The purpose of this chapter has been to review possible legal bases for physician liability in TD litigation and to provide specific clinical guidelines for practice. Possibly the best protection from litigation is good clinical practice, maintaining good working relationships with patients, taking time to discuss their concerns, and remaining sensitive to their rights in the decision-making process.

REFERENCES

1. Black HC: Black's Law Dictionary. St Paul, MN, West Publishing, 1986

2. Prosser W: Handbook of the Law of Torts (fourth edition). St Paul, MN, West Publishing, 1971

3. Shapiro SA: Limiting physician freedom to prescribe a drug for any purpose: the need for FDA regulation. Northwestern University Law Review 73:801–872, 1979

4. Wettstein RM, Appelbaum PS: Legal liability for tardive dyskinesia. Hosp Community Psychiatry 35:992–993, 1984

5. Freishtat HW: Forensic update: view from the nation's courts. J Clin Psychopharmacol 3:49–50, 1983

6. Wettstein RM: Tardive dyskinesia and malpractice. Behavioral Science and the Law 1:85–107, 1983

7. Taub S: Tardive dyskinesia: medical facts and legal fictions. St Louis University Law Journal 30:833-873, 1986

8. Flaherty JA, Channon R, David J (eds): Clinical Manual of Psychiatric Therapeutics. East Norwolk, CT, Appleton-Century-Crofts (in press)

9. Gutheil TG, Appelbaum PS: Clinical Handbook of Psychiatry and the Law. New York, McGraw-Hill Book, 1982

10. Mills MJ, Norquist GS, Shelton RC, et al: Consent and liability with neuroleptics: the problems of tardive dyskinesia. International Journal of Law and Psychiatry 8:243–252, 1986

11. Munetz MR: Overcoming resistance to talking to patients about tardive dyskinesia. Hosp Community Psychiatry 36:283–287, 1985

12. DeVeaugh-Geiss J: Informed consent for neuroleptic therapy. Am J Psychiatry 136:959–962, 1979

13. Jaffe R: Problems of long-term informed consent. Bulletin of the American Academy of Psychiatry and the Law 14:163–169, 1986

14. Ganguli R, Raghu U: Tardive dyskinesia, impaired recall, and informed consent. J Clin Psychiatry 46:434–435, 1985

15. Munetz MR, Roth LH: Informing patients about tardive dyskinesia. Arch Gen Psychiatry 42:866–871, 1985

16. McClellan FM: Strict liability for drug induced injuries: an excursion through the maze of products liability, negligence and absolute liability. Wayne University Law Review 25:2–36, 1978

17. Appelbaum PS, Schaffner K, Meisel A: Responsibility and compensation for tardive dyskinesia. Am J Psychiatry 142:806–810, 1985

18. Moore RM: Consent forms—how, or whether, they should be used. Mayo Clin Proc 53:393–396, 1978

19. Glazer WM: Informed consent. Psychiatric News, November 1984

20. Munetz MR, Roth LH, Cornes CL: Tardive dyskinesia and informed consent: myths and realities. Bulletin of the American Academy of Psychiatry and the Law 10:77–88, 1982

21. Task Force on Late Neurological Effects of Antipsychotic Drugs: Tardive dyskinesia: summary of a task force report of the American Psychiatric Association. Am J Psychiatry 137:1163–1172, 1980

22. Sovner R, DiMascio A, Berkowitz D, et al: Tardive dyskinesia and informed consent. Psychosomatics 19:172–177, 1978

23. Gualtieri CT, Barnhill J, McGimsey J, et al: Tardive dyskinesia and other movement disorders in children treated with psychotropic drugs. J Am Acad Child Psychiatry 19:491–510, 1980

24. Gualtieri CT, Breuning SE, Schroeder SR, et al: Tardive dyskinesia in mentally retarded children, adolescents, and young adults: North Carolina and Michigan studies. Psychopharmacol Bull 18:62–65, 1982

25. May PRA, Tuma AH, Dixon WJ: Schizophrenia: a follow-up study of the results of five forms of treatment. Arch Gen Psychiatry 38:776–784, 1981

26. Stone AA: The new paradox of psychiatric malpractice. N Engl J Med 311:1384–1387, 1984

27. Epstein LC, Lasagna L: Obtaining informed consent. Arch Intern Med 123:682–688, 1969

28. Ayd FJ: Ethical and legal dilemmas posed by the tardive dyskinesia. International Drug Therapy Newsletter 12(8 & 9):29–36, 1977

29. Goldman MB, Luchins DJ: Intermittent neuroleptic therapy and tardive dyskinesia: a literature review. Hosp Community Psychiatry 35:1215–1219, 1984

30. Gualtieri CT, Sprague RL, Cole JO: Tardive dyskinesia litigation and the dilemmas of neuroleptic treatment. Journal of Psychiatry and Law 14:187–216, 1986

31. Jeste DV, Potkin SG, Sinha S, et al: Tardive dyskinesia—reversible and persistent. Arch Gen Psychiatry 36:585–590, 1979

32. Pyke J, Seeman MN: Neuroleptic-free intervals in the treatment of schizophrenia. Am J Psychiatry 138:1620–1621, 1981

33. Olson GW, Peterson OB: Intermittent chemotherapy for chronic psychiatric inpatients. J Nerv Ment Dis 134:145–149, 1962

34. Johnson DAW: Antipsychotic medication: clinical guidelines for maintenance therapy. J Clin Psychiatry 46(5, Sec 2):6–15, 1985

35. Whall AL, Engle V, Edwards A, et al: Development of a screening program for tardive dyskinesia: feasibility issues. Nurs Res 32:151–156, 1983

36. Munetz MR, Schulz SC. Screening for tardive dyskinesia. J Clin Psychiatry 47:75–77, 1986

NOTES

1. *Clites v. Iowa*, 322 NW2d 917 (Iowa App 1982).

2. *Faigenbaum v. Oakland Medical Center*, 373 NW2d 161 (Mich App 1985).

3. *Lundgren v. Eustermann*, 370 NW2d 877 (Minn 1985).

4. *Hedin v. United States*, No. 5-83-3, Slip op (D Minn Jan 4, 1985).

5. See *Lundgren v. Eustermann*, supra note 3, at 880.

6. *Helling v. Carey*, 519 P2d 981 (83 Wash 2d 246) 1979.

7. See also *Gates v. Jensen*, 595 P2d 919 (92 Wash 2d 246) 1979.

8. *Salgo v. Leland Stanford Jr. University*, 317 P2d, 170, 181 (Cal 1957).

9. *Canterbury v. Spence*, 464 F2d 772 (DC Cir 1972).

10. See also *Truman v. Thomas*, 611 P2d 902 (Cal 1980).

11. *Barclay v. Campbell*, 704 SW2d 8 (Tex 1986).

12. Id. at 11.

13. *Guilmet v. Campbell*, 188 NW2d 601 (Mich 1971).

14. *Johnston v. Rodis*, 251 F2d 917 (DC Cir 19589).

15. *Simcuski v. Saeli*, 377 NE2d 713, 406 NYS2d 259 (1978).

16. *Sandoz, Inc. v. Employer's Liability Assurance Corporation*, 554 F Supp 257 (D C N J 1983).

17. *Helling v. Carey*, supra note 6.

18. *Gates v. Jensen*, supra note 7.

19. See, e.g., *Rogers v. Okin*, 478 F Supp 1342 (D Mass 1979), aff'd in part, rev'd in part, vacated and remanded, 634 F2d 630 (1st Cir 1980), vacated and remanded sub nom *Mills v. Rogers*, 457 US 291 (1982).

20. See, e.g., *Rennie v. Klein*, 653 F2d 836 (3rd Cir 1981); 720 F2d 266 (3rd Cir 1983). The *Rennie* court reasoned that a patient's constitutional right to refuse antipsychotic medications depends upon whether he is a danger to himself or others, as determined by professional judgment.

21. See, e.g., *Stensvad v. Reivitz*, 601 F Supp 128 (WD Wisc 1985).

22. See, e.g., *In re Roe III*, 421 NE 2d 40 (Mass 1981); *People v. Medina*, 705 P2d 961 (Colo 1985).

23. *Cathmer v. Hunter*, 558 P2d 975 (27 Ariz App 780) 1976.

24. *Siegel v. Mount Sinai Hospital of Cleveland*, 403 NE2d 202 (62 Ohio App 2d 12) 1978.

25. *Tunk v. Regents of the University of California*, 383 P2d 441 (32 Cal Rptr 33) 1963.

26. Supra, note 4.

27. Supra, note 1.

28. This summary is a synthesis of the Task Force guidelines as described in the following sources: American Psychiatric Association Task Force on Late Neurological Effects of Antipsychotic Drugs, Tardive Dyskinesia, Task Force Report 18. Washington, DC, American Psychiatric Association, 1979; Tardive dyskinesia: summary of a task force report of the American Psychiatric Association. Am J Psychiatry 137:1163–1172, 1980; letter from American Psychiatric Association to American Psychiatric Association members (July 1985); Summary on tardive dyskinesia, Psychiatric News, May 17, 1985, p. 7.

Chapter 19

Overcoming Institutional and Community Resistance to a Tardive Dyskinesia Management Program

Marion E. Wolf, M.D.
Phil Brown, Ph.D.

Chapter 19

Overcoming Institutional and Community Resistance to a Tardive Dyskinesia Management Program

Tardive dyskinesia is an involuntary movement disorder caused by prolonged neuroleptic treatment. The prevalence rate of tardive dyskinesia has increased over time and is now estimated at 26 percent (1). Many consider tardive dyskinesia a public health concern.

Although there was significant evidence of the tardive dyskinesia problem as early as the 1960s, most clinicians were not aware of it (2). Clinicians' failure to adequately recognize the problem may have stemmed from their difficulty in evaluating clinically useful drugs in a critical manner; difficulty in accepting responsibility for an iatrogenic illness; insufficient appreciation of the patient's experience of side effects; and fear that dealing openly with tardive dyskinesia will lead to treatment refusal and clinical decompensation (2–5).

The 1979 American Psychiatric Association (APA) Task Force Report on late neurological effects of antipsychotic drugs was a significant response to the problem of tardive dyskinesia (6). The report recommended careful monitoring for side effects of antipsychotic drugs, judicious use of antipsychotic agents, discussion with patients and their families about the benefits and risks of neuroleptic

This chapter is reprinted with permission from *Hospital and Community Psychiatry* 38:65–68, 1987 (copyright 1987 American Psychiatric Association).

The authors wish to express their sincere thanks to Jochnan Wolf, M.D., Ross Baldessarini, M.D., George Simpson, M.D., and Robert Sprague, Ph.D.

use, and withdrawal or reduction in dose of the antipsychotic agent upon discovery of tardive dyskinesia symptoms. Few institutions have adopted the APA guidelines, and in those that have, many professionals try to circumvent them (7, 8). Even when informed consent about psychiatric treatment is seriously pursued, patients are provided little information about side effects (9). When side effects are mentioned, tardive dyskinesia is frequently not among those named (10).

Despite common fears to the contrary, experience indicates that informing patients about the risks of tardive dyskinesia does not lead to treatment refusal, clinical decompensation, rehospitalization, or litigation (11). However, several malpractice cases concerning tardive dyskinesia have been decided for large sums, based mainly on the clinician's failure to warn patients and families about the risks of tardive dyskinesia (12).

Several investigators have reported resistance among psychiatrists toward implementation of measures aimed at the prevention and management of tardive dyskinesia (2–5, 7, 8, 13). Little has been said, however, about the resistance of nursing staff, institutions, and communities to dealing with tardive dyskinesia. This chapter describes social issues that were addressed during the implementation of the APA task force guidelines on tardive dyskinesia on an inpatient unit and in an outpatient setting.

The guidelines were implemented by the tardive dyskinesia program at the North Chicago Veterans Administration (V.A.) Medical Center. The program consists of both clinical and research sections. The clinical section provides consultation, evaluation, and treatment for patients with tardive dyskinesia in an inpatient unit, where patients stay for 30 days. The research section is concerned with implementation of research protocols. The program was developed in 1980 with the strong support of hospital officials.

IMPLEMENTATION ON AN INPATIENT UNIT

The attempt to implement the APA guidelines on the tardive dyskinesia unit was met with resistance by the nursing staff, which proved to be a significant problem. The nurses were opposed to instituting drug-free periods for patients on chronic neuroleptic therapy, as recommended in the APA guidelines. The patients' neuroleptic doses were progressively reduced until the patients were no longer taking the neuroleptics, after which they remained drug free for 2 weeks.

The program staff conducted many extra meetings and workshops to convince staff on all shifts that this intervention was medically sound, safe, and feasible. Staff feared and expected that patients would experience clinical decompensation. They also feared an increase in "incident reports," which could be viewed as reflections of poor care and could even lead to litigation if the incidents were severe.

In the beginning staff considered any change in a patient's behavior during drug discontinuation as an indication of deterioration. However, after repeated drug-free periods, staff learned that patients rarely became assaultive or even posed a significant management problem. Furthermore, some patients improved when excessive doses of neuroleptics were discontinued. The direct involvement of clinical staff of the tardive dyskinesia program in drug-free periods and in staff education, as well as the benefit of experience, gradually changed the staff's view. The clear lesson is that a concerned program to address tardive dyskinesia can succeed, even though initial opposition and fear may hinder its start-up.

IMPLEMENTATION IN AN OUTPATIENT SETTING

In 1985 the tardive dyskinesia program staff were asked to evaluate and treat tardive dyskinesia among patients in the V.A. Medical Center's community care placement program. Unlike working with the inpatient unit, working in the outpatient setting required that program staff deal with factors not under their control. A factor of particular interest was the community sponsors' opposition to reduction in patients' psychotropic medication.

The community care placement program provides care for 168 discharged chronic psychiatric patients who live in the private homes of nonprofessional community sponsors. The sponsors are under contract with the V.A. to provide the patients' meals, supervise their medication, and take them to doctors' appointments at the community care placement clinic at the V.A. medical center.

The program staff evaluated every patient who visited the community care placement clinic over a 2-month period, a total of 76 patients. The clinical characteristics of the patients are described in Table 1. The patients received neuropsychiatric evaluations and were scored on Simpson's tardive dyskinesia rating scale (14). No veteran refused to be evaluated.

All the patients had been or were currently receiving neuroleptics, and 40, or 52.6 percent, were found to have tardive dyskinesia. Neuroleptic medication was discontinued or the dosage decreased in 63 percent of the patients with tardive dyskinesia. Antiparkinsonian drugs were discontinued in 83 percent of the patients with tardive dyskinesia. Table 2 summarizes patients' use of medication before and after the intervention of the program staff.

Most patients accepted the program staff's explanations of the reasons for changes in their medication. However, their community sponsors responded by increasing by 50 percent the patients' un-scheduled visits to the clinic, by increasing by 30 percent the patients' after-hours visits to a cooperating V.A. mental health clinic, and by making repeated telephone calls to request additional psychotropic medication for the patients.

During visits by staff to patients and their sponsors at home, the sponsors expressed fears that the loss of medication would undermine the stability of the patients whose medication was reduced as well as that of other patients under their care. The sponsors were reassured that the community care placement clinic would follow patients closely, that negative outcomes were not expected, and that their role in the patients' care was considered essential.

Subsequently the staff organized educational activities for the sponsors, conducted at the V.A. medical center. As part of the activities, the effects and problems of psychotropic drugs and the efficacy of moderate doses of neuroleptics were discussed in plain language (15). The educational activities appeared to facilitate the smooth operation of the program, suggesting that consideration of social issues may reduce pressure on physicians to revert to often excessive neuroleptic prescriptions to avoid difficulties arising from changes in treatment.

Table 1. Clinical characteristics of 76 patients in a community care placement program.

Characteristic	n	%
Tardive dyskinesia	40	52.6
No tardive dyskinesia	36	47.4
Primary psychiatric diagnosis		
Schizophrenia	41	54.0
Affective disorder	28	36.8
Organic mental disorder	4	5.3
Other	3	4.0
Secondary psychiatric diagnosis		
Alcoholism	17	22.4
Organic mental disorder	6	7.9
Personality disorder	8	10.5
Other	2	2.6
Concurrent medical diagnosis	43	56.6
Two or more concurrent medical diagnoses	13	17.1

Table 2. Use of medications by 40 patients with tardive dyskinesia before and after intervention by tardive dyskinesia program staff.

Medication	Before intervention		After intervention	
	n	%	n	%
Neuroleptics	30	75.0	11[a]	27.5
Antiparkinsonian agents	12	30.0	2	5.0
Lithium	9	22.5	10	25.0
Antidepressants	3	7.5	2	5.0
Carbamazepine	3	7.5	3	7.5
Other anticonvulsants	1	2.5	1	2.5

[a]Includes only patients whose neuroleptic dose after intervention was similar to or higher than their dose before intervention.

INSTITUTIONAL OBSTACLES

Psychiatric hospitals are composed of different constituents with various goals (16, 17). Therefore innovations require some consensus among groups. Implementation of changes aimed at the prevention and management of tardive dyskinesia at our medical center required concerted efforts from different services such as psychiatry, psychology, nursing, social work, and pharmacy. It also necessitated the development of better means of communication between different programs, such as the community care placement clinic and the V.A.'s day treatment program. Several patients in the community care placement program also attended the day treatment program, requiring that staff of the day treatment program be involved in changes in the patients' chemotherapy.

Implementation of the tardive dyskinesia guidelines produced greater demands on the clinic physician's time. The physician's increased responsibilities included conducting thorough, multiple evaluations of the patients for tardive dyskinesia, teaching therapeutic effects and side effects of psychotropic drugs to staff and community care placement sponsors, and carrying out added administrative tasks, for example, attending more administrative meetings.

The tardive dyskinesia program staff found that institutional obstacles did not halt or seriously hinder the program's activities. Nevertheless, staff felt pressure to maintain the status quo. The 1979 American Psychiatric Association Task Force on tardive dyskinesia addressed the issue of resistance to discontinuation of neuroleptics in chronically hospitalized patients, stating that "the potential benefits outweigh the possible risks and the natural reluctance of those caring for fairly stable chronically ill patients to rock the boat" (6).

Thus, to implement a tardive dyskinesia program, it is necessary to overcome institutional inertia. Furthermore, institutional leadership is also required to obtain support for allocating mental health professionals trained in effective screening for tardive dyskinesia as well as to obtain funds for education of staff, patients, families, and community members.

The development of a program for the prevention and management of tardive dyskinesia may result in initial budgetary increases. In light of that, it is important to note Kalachnik's calculation (18) that a thorough tardive dyskinesia screening program for a 4,000-bed system over a period of 17 and a half years would be equivalent to the typical cost of one plaintiff's successful malpractice litigation. In any case, concern for the patients' well-being, not financial considerations alone, should be the central factor when formulating policy.

CONCLUSION

Community and institutional barriers make it difficult to implement programs for screening and treatment of tardive dyskinesia that meet the APA Task Force's recommendations for sound practice. Concerted efforts at liaison with and education for staff, communities, and institutions can reduce such opposition. It is important that high-level administrative leadership be behind such efforts. If multiple institutions develop tardive dyskinesia programs, more mental health professionals will be made aware of the clinical and professional benefits of such programs and will therefore be more accepting of them.

REFERENCES

1. Jeste DV, Wyatt RJ: Understanding and Treating Tardive Dyskinesia. New York, Guilford Press, 1982

2. Crane GE: The prevention of tardive dyskinesia. Am J Psychiatry 134:756–758, 1977

3. Brown P, Funk SC: Tardive dyskinesia: barriers to the recognition of an iatrogenic disease. J Health Soc Behav 27:116–132, 1986

4. Paulson GW: Tardive dyskinesia. Annual Review of Medicine 25:75–80, 1975

5. Munetz MR: Overcoming resistance to talking to patients about tardive dyskinesia. Hosp Community Psychiatry 36:283–287, 1985

6. Baldessarini RJ, Cole JD, David JM, et al: Report of the American Psychiatric Association Task Force on Late Neurological Effects of Antipsychotic Drugs. Washington, DC, American Psychiatric Association, 1979

7. Gualtieri CT, Sprague RL: Preventing tardive dyskinesia and preventing tardive dyskinesia legislation. Psychopharmacol Bull 20:346–348, 1984

8. Munetz MR, Roth LH, Cornes CL: Tardive dyskinesia and informed consent: myths and realities. Bulletin of the American Academy of Psychiatry and the Law 10:77–88, 1982

9. Lidz CW, Meisel A, Zerubavel E, et al: Informed Consent: A Study of Decision Making in Psychiatry. New York, Guilford Press, 1983

10. Benson PR: Informed consent: drug information disclosed to patients prescribed antipsychotic medication. J Nerv Ment Dis 172:642–653, 1984

11. Munetz MR, Roth LH: Informing patients about tardive dyskinesia. Arch Gen Psychiatry 42:866–871, 1985

12. Sprague RL: Litigation, legislation, and regulations, in Drugs and Mental Retardation. Edited by Breuning SE, Poling AD. Springfield, IL, Thomas, 1982

13. Glazer W, Moore DC: A tardive dyskinesia clinic in a mental health center. Hosp Community Psychiatry 32:572–574, 1981

14. Simpson GM, Lee JH, Zoubok B, et al: A rating scale for tardive dyskinesia. Psychopharmacology 64:171–179, 1985

15. Teicher MH, Baldessarini RJ: Selection of neuroleptic dosage. Arch Gen Psychiatry 42:636–637, 1985

16. Perrow C: Complex Organizations: A Critical Essay. Glenview, IL, Scott Foresman, 1979

17. Strauss A, Schatzman L, Bucher R, et al: Psychiatric Ideologies and Institutions. New York, Free Press, 1964

18. Kalachnik JE: Beyond Chicken Wire and Spit: A Tardive Dyskinesia Monitoring System for Applied Facilities (NTIS Publication PB85-109171). Springfield, VA, U.S. Department of Commerce, 1984